Return on or before the
last date stamped below.

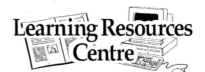

D1343583

Iris Pahmeier/Corinna Niederbäumer

Step Aerobics

Fitness Training for Schools, Clubs and Studios

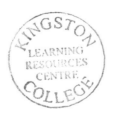

KINGSTON
LEARNING
RESOURCES
CENTRE
COLLEGE

Meyer & Meyer Sport

Original title:
Step-Aerobic für Schule, Verein und Studio
4. Auflage – Aachen: Meyer und Meyer Verlag, 2000

British Library Cataloguing in Publication Data
A catalogue for this book is available from the British Library

Pahmeier / Niederbäumer
Step Aerobics/ Iris Pahmeier; Corinna Niederbäumer.
– Oxford: Meyer & Meyer Sport (UK) Ltd., 2001
ISBN 1-84126-025-8

All rights reserved. Expect for use in a review, no part of this publication may be
reproduced, stored in a retrieval system, or transmitted, in any form or by any
means now known or hereafter invented without the prior written permission
of the publisher. This book may not be lent, resold, hired out or otherwise
disposed of by way of trade in any form, binding or cover other than that which
is published, without the prior written consent of the publisher.

© 2001 by Meyer & Meyer Sport (UK) Ltd.
Oxford, Aachen, Olten (CH), Vienna, Québec, Lansing/Michigan, Adelaide,
Auckland, Johannesburg, Budapest
Member of the World
Sport Publishers' Association (WSPA)
www.w-s-p-a.org

Cover Photo: Sportpressefoto Bongarts, Hamburg
Photos: Christoph Brütting, Pottenstein
Illustrations: Heike Ullrich, Frankfurt a. Main; Ines Walter, Bayreuth
Cover design: Birgit Engelen, Stolberg
Cover and type exposure: frw, Reiner Wahlen, Aachen
Editorial: John Coghlan, Michelle Dull
Printed and bound in Germany
by Burgverlag Gastinger GmbH, Stolberg
ISBN 1-84126-025-8
e-mail: verlag@meyer-meyer-sports.com
www.meyer-meyer-sports.com

KING'S COLLEGE
LEARNING RESOURCES CENTRE

Class No. 796·04 PAH

Acc. No. 00136747

Date Rec. 11/05

Order No. 734450

Contents

● ● ● ● ●

Throughout this book, the pronouns he, she, him, her and so on are interchangeable and intended to be inclusive of both men and women. It is important in sport, as elsewhere, that men and women have equal status and opportunities.

Introduction

Step aerobics is the most successful trend in the area of commercial fitness since the appearance of the aerobics craze in the early 1980s. At the beginning of the 90s, Step aerobics was introduced into Europe to continue its success boom there. Current observations indicate that fashionable trends are increasingly finding their way into established sports organisations, and they are not the only ones opening up to these new opportunities. Sports education in schools is also being influenced by new kinds of sport and fitness trends. In contrast to established kinds of sport and fitness activities which are discussed in the press, committed teachers, trainers and exercise leaders who wish to teach step aerobics are faced with a striking deficit as there are few specialists avaible on the subject. Knowledge is marketed internally and at a high price on the commercial fitness scene, in workshops, via training sessions or on videos.

This book aims to offer further assistance. It has been conceived as a practical book aimed at teachers, exercise leaders and sports instructors who teach step aerobics in various institutions or those who are interested in more ways of using step apparatus in fitness and health training.

In order to be able to offer step aerobics, it is necessary to understand and describe the content and techniques of this sport. One must also have complete knowledge of the appropriate teaching methods so that all the step patterns and arm movements are put together and mastered in such a way that the participants do not have any interruption to their workout. An understanding of programme structure with varying emphases in training, and varying target groups (beginners, intermediate and advanced), ensures, moreover, a motivating and appealing training organisation. The aim of this book is to inform the reader about some of these aspects and to offer a few practical ideas.

To achieve this the book is divided into two sections. The first three chapters are on theory and present an overview of origins, aims, training possibilities and step aerobics programmes. The results of research already done in the sport of step aerobics are summarized in chapter two. Chapter three concentrates exclusively on teaching methods.

In the extensive practical section the reader is informed about the techniques of step aerobics. This comprises a detailed description of basic steps, step combinations, arm movements and patterns. These techniques are presented in the standard language of this sport. The section on technique is rounded off with a description of strength and flexibility exercises with the step apparatus. These are followed by suggestions for an alternative, playful use of the step apparatus. The five practical examples given in chapter five enable those interested to construct their own programmes for teaching and step training. At the end you will find two further teaching ideas for use in school sports.

1 Step Aerobics: Fitness Training for Schools, Clubs and Studios

Step aerobics is a form of fitness training done to music with a right-angled platform where the height can be varied. Training is characterized by the various ways of stepping on and off this platform with different kinds of arm movements.

Gin Miller is seen as the inventor of step aerobics. After injuring her knee, she was prescribed a course of physiotherapy during rehabilitation for training her thigh muscles back to normal. This programme involved stepping on and off a medium-high box. To take the monotony out of her training, Gin Miller set it to music and went on to develop different kinds of step patterns and combined these with arm movements. The basic concept of step aerobics was thus born.

Reebok, the manufacturer of sporting products, took hold of the idea and promoted one of the most successful fitness trends of recent years – the "Step-Reebok-Programme". Alongside the development of the sports apparatus „Step-Reebok", the marketing company also produced exercise activities on the step apparatus.

Kelly Watson and Gin Miller are seen as the source of this creativity. They launched the steps, step patterns, arm movements and choreography for the programmes. A further important move of Reebok was their scientific safeguarding of the programme, for which the American sports and fitness experts, Dr. Peter Francis and Dr. Lorna Francis were engaged. All previous theoretical and practical knowledge was put together in a written training manual which was given to everyone who completed the Reebok instructor's course.

Since the introduction of step aerobics in America in the early 80s, this form of fitness training has enjoyed continuous popularity in fitness and aerobics circles. It has been estimated that in the U.S.A. alone over 9 Million people practise step training regularly. Step training also takes up 50% of all aerobic courses (see RIPPE 1994). Since the beginning of the

90s this trend has been successfully continued in Europe in the area of commercial fitness. The undoubted success of the sport step aerobics cannot totally rest on the attraction of step aerobics itself, or on skilled marketing strategy. There must already be fertile ground for such a seed.

Even if the aerobics movement appeared to have died in the middle of the previous decade, it experienced its renaissance in the early 90s. Fitness and aerobic activities are currently the fastest growing forms of workout amongst adults. In Germany, for example, a representative survey published by the Institute of Leisure Science in 1993 confirms this trend with some impressive figures. About 3.7 million people take part regularly once a week in clubs, fitness courses, as well as 1.4 million in other courses, mainly at fitness studios. 3.2 million Germans currently train at least once a week on fitness apparatus. A 250% rate of increase was observed in this area in recent years.

Also in non-profit organizations, i.e. in the traditional sports clubs, the most significant rates of increase have been noted mainly on what is offered in the areas of gymnastics, health and fitness (see HEINEMANN/ SCHUBERT 1994). In addition to this, similar activities are being offered in the areas of health and education. Universities and health insurance firms are among the main suppliers (see BREHM 1995).

There are many reasons for such a boom: a changed attitude towards one's health due to increased awareness has made the population sensitive to detrimental influences. In large sectors of the population one can see an increased willingness to change one's lifestyle, and this is where doing some kind of sport begins.

Certain types of gymnastics, fitness activities and aerobics for beginners or those starting again are particularly suitable because these activities guarantee an all-round improvement to quality of life. These include strengthening one's level of physical fitness, improving physical and mental resilience and vitality, improving one's appearance, and experiencing emotional stability and a feeling of general wellbeing. Young adults in particular have so far been responsive to this offer. About 50%

of the participants are aged between 20 and 30 and a further 20% between 30 and 40 (see BRETTSCHNEIDER/ BRÄUTIGAM 1990; KAMBEROVIC/ HASE 1994). Likewise in sports clubs, the vast increase in fitness training offered can be attributed to the increasing demand and participation of adults over 20. At the same time, adult women in particular feel drawn to fitness programmes and their participation percentage is well over 50%.

Even the traditional sports organizations have not closed their eyes to addressing new target groups with the aim of making themselves members. Also when discussions take place about the up-to-date content of school sports, a lot of intensive debate goes on as to how to bring modern sport and fitness trends into practice (see BALZ a.o. 1994, SCHULZ 1994).

A final reason concerns aerobics itself. In recent years this kind of sport has seen a change for the better due to approval from the sports medicine and scientific training angle as well as an accompanying change of content. At the moment one can also see more professionalism in teaching methods, which is another important aspect when recommending this sport for schools, clubs and studios.

1.1 The Origin of Step Aerobics

The origin of step aerobics is clearly to be found in general aerobics, which in their turn originated with the American sports doctor, Kenneth H. Cooper, the undisputed founder of the endurance movement. Since the 60s Cooper has prescribed and upheld this preventative creed. At that time, while working for the U.S. Air Force, he developed an endurance training programme for NASA astronauts to economize their cardiac work. The programme consisted of endurance sports like running, cycling and swimming, which he called "aerobics" (Greek aer = air), because they boost the turnover of oxygen in the body. This sparked a fitness boom in the U.S.A. and made the doctor famous all over the world.

The founders of the aerobics movement have taken up this aspect of aerobic endurance training, namely maintaining the use of the larger groups of muscles over an extended period of time, in order to stimulate the heart and circulatory system.

At the same time, ideas from the world of gymnastics and dance spread into this new form of fitness. Jackie Sorensen has devised a programme of 30 minutes of endurance training followed by exercises for muscle strengthening which she calls "isotonics" (see SORENSEN 1983). Judy Sheppard-Missed combines aerobics with advanced co-ordination exercises and elements of jazz-dance (see SHEPPARD-MISSED 1986). Jane Fonda combines aerobics endurance training with gymnastic exercises for strength endurance and flexibility in her "Workout Programme", all of which is performed to a musical rhythm (see FONDA 1983). Aerobic fever was also started by an actress in Germany. At the beginning of the 1980s, Sidney Rome popularized this form of fitness training (see ROME 1983).

Due to the indiscriminate and somewhat careless transfer of aerobic movement patterns, this kind of sport soon drifted onto the sidelines in other countries such as Germany. It was regarded as non-functional and untenable from a physical training point of view, and justifiably received massive criticism from sports scientists and sports doctors. One of the main reasons for the sport of aerobics to be given a second chance in Germany can attributed to the work of the "German Aerobics Association" (DAV).

This association was founded more or less at the same time as the collapse of public enthusiasm in Germany for the first craze, and it now aims to extend aerobic sports. The DAV has also devised a training concept with a final aerobics instructor's certificate based on sports medicine, didactic and methodic knowledge (research). Thus, at the start of the 90s, the second aerobics craze hit Germany, showing two new tendencies compared with the first boom. First, increased scientific training and knowledge of sports medicine are incorporated in the training process. Second, the choreography is prepared and transmitted according to specific teaching methods (see DAV 1993).

Since 1993, aerobics has been an official competitive type of sport under the auspices of the German Gymnasts' Association (Deutscher Turner-Bund, DTB). Since 1994 the association has also offered their own aerobics training instruction for popular and leisure sport, which has been well received by exercise leaders. Overall, 400 DTB aerobics trainers have qualified so far in 13 basic training courses. From 1996 onwards there will be a corresponding training course for step aerobics (see DTB 1993, 1994 and 1995).

Any careful observer of the fast-moving fitness scene of today could get the impression that one trend is chasing another. However, on closer inspection it can be seen that permanent and well-defined motor or technical performance elements, e.g. arm and leg movements, have been developed for aerobics sport and its various branches. There are fixed programme sequences, music is now an indispensable component of every aerobics class and compulsory teaching methods are now being established.

Step aerobics has benefited from these developments as well as the addition of significant aspects from general aerobics.

1.2 Step Aerobics as Fitness Training

FITNESS	
Health-orientated fitness	*Sport-orientated fitness*
• Aerobic endurance	• Anaerobic endurance
• Strength endurance	• Resilience, explosive strength, maximum strength, reactive strength
• Optimum flexibility	• Speed, speed endurance
• Psychological and physical ability to relax	• Maximum flexibility (hyperflexibility)
• Healthy diet, optimum body composition	
• General co-ordination ability	• Special co-ordination ability, sport-oriented techniques

Diagram 1: Fitness factors (according to: BOECKH-BEHRENS/ BUSKIES 1995, 15)

Step aerobics is an all-embracing kind of fitness training. Fitness and wellness are key words that are now closely bound with popular and leisure sport. Whereas the term "fitness" originally had a wide meaning, it became confined to physical factors in the mid-70s so that fitness referred exclusively to a person's endurance performance potential. At present, the word is being extended again. In everyday language, so maintains WOPP (1995, 122) "Fitness refers to physical and mental health". Other authors, however, differentiate between health-oriented fitness and sports fitness (see BOECKH-BEHRENS/ BUSKIES 1995).

Following the above differentiation, (see diagram 1, p. 13) Step aerobics training should address the fitness components of aerobic endurance, strength flexibility and one's general co-ordinative skill. The prime aim is to have a positive effect on one's physical, and above all, one's psychological wellbeing.

1.2.1 Fitness Training Is Endurance Training

Step aerobics promises to train general dynamic endurance and thus to maintain or improve the functioning of the heart and circulatory system.

The word "endurance" means, on the whole, resilience to psychological and physical tiredness (see WEINECK 1990), i.e. the ability to maintain physical exertion over a longer period of time. There is a general demand put on dynamic and aerobic endurance, when 1/6 to 1/7 of the whole skeletal muscles is being used, whilst using more than 50% of the maximum heart and circulation potential.

How can I train my endurance?

In order to improve general aerobic endurance potential, dynamic use of the larger groups of muscles must take place. This happens when jogging, swimming, walking, skiing, rowing and training with endurance apparatus, aerobics and step aerobics. These activities should be done by putting between 50-70% load on the circulatory system's maximum potential.

Duration of load or stress should be maintained for at least ten minutes (see DE MAREES 1987). At best the stress load should not exceed 30 or 40 minutes, as then not only cardiopulmonary but also metabolic signs of adaptability take place in the organ system (see HOLLMANN/ HETTINGER 1990). Training should be done at least twice a week, throughout life, to maintain endurance level.

How can I control my use of stamina?

Pulse taking should be established in training sessions in order to ascertain the stress intensity when doing sport and also to best regulate and guide individual stress levels. A guide to individual heart rates for training can be taken from charts, which take three factors into consideration when calculating the appropriate stress level: age, resting heart rate and type of endurance activity.

The optimum training heart rate, i.e. the number of heart beats per minute that one should have after running and doing aerobics or step aerobics, can be read from the chart below.

Resting heart rate in 15 seconds ↓	Age →Under 30	30-39	40-49	50-59	60-70	Over 70
Under 13	35	35	34	33	31	30
13-14	35	35	34	33	31	30
15-17	36	36	35	34	33	31
18-20	36	36	35	34	33	31
20-22	38	36	35	34	33	31
23-25	38	38	36	35	34	33
Over 25	39	38	36	36	35	33

Chart 1: A guide to heart rate levels for beginning runners (modified according to LAGERSTROEM 1983)

In more recent times, feeling exertion as a measure of stress intensity has overridden the criterion of recording heart rate. The person in training registers his subjectively felt level of exertion and regulates its intensity accordingly. For example, if a V-step with arm movements is seen to be too taxing, then the trainee can just continue the step pattern without the arms. Subjective stress sensitivity can also be measured. The BORG RPE Scale (1985) has proved helpful and practical for this. RPE Scale means "scale for ratings (R) of perceived (P) exertion (E)". The subsequently developed scale of exertion (see BREHM/ PAHMEIER/ TIEMANN 1994) is shown in the next diagram:

Exertion Measurement Scale:

6	no exertion at all
7	very, very slight
8	
9	very slight
10	
11	slight
12	**this is your ideal**
13	a bit more intense **training area**
14	
15	considerable
16	
17	intense
18	
19	extremely intense
20	the maximum amount of exertion

Diagram 2: Exertion Measurement Scale (following the BORG RPE Scale 1985,7)

This measurement scale ranging from 6 (minimum exertion) to 20 (maximum exertion) comprises 15 exertion levels with which the exertion felt can be differentiated and estimated. A favourable level of exertion both from a physical and psychological point of view happens when one's feeling of exertion lies within the 11-14 range during step training, i.e. the trainee feels slightly to a bit more intensely stretched (see BUSKIES/ KLÄGER/ RIEDEL 1992).

What causes good stamina?

Training endurance regularly leads to improved co-ordination and flexibility. Endurance training particularly affects the heart and circulatory system. The heart beats more slowly because it can pump more blood with each beat than an untrained heart can. The body has a better supply of blood and nutrients because they are supplied in the pauses between beats, which become longer the slower the heart beats. The heart adjusts more quickly to exertion and thus has greater reserves.

This is a positive secondary benefit to one's physical and emotional state of health. On a physical level in particular it has a positive effect on the risk factors of high blood pressure, raised blood fat level as well as raised blood sugar level.

Possible coronary heart disease, arteriosclerosis and diabetes are also counteracted. In addition, one can help prevent obesity by endurance training. It has also been proved that the higher the endurance level of a human being, the more resilient he is emotionally. He feels better able to cope with stress and is more psychologically stable.

1.2.2 Fitness Training Is Strength Training

Step aerobics promises to improve strength, and above all, to maintain or improve one's structure and posture.

The word strength or power means the ability to overcome resistance by tensing the muscles, or the ability to counteract resistance by giving way or maintaining resistance. Good strength is not only the basis for all muscular movement, but also guarantees good body posture. A person who does not train his strength between age of 20 and 70 loses 30-40% of his muscle structure, and at the same time the quality of the muscle cells deteriorates.

How can I train strength?

Static and dynamic methods can be implemented to improve strength potential. During static strength training, the muscles are tensed against a fixed object, e.g. one's own body, a partner, strength training equipment or other materials. The intensity of tension must reach 30% of the individual's muscle power. The optimum level is at an intensity between 50 - 70%. Static strengthening exercises are especially recommended for training the trunk muscles, as these have a stationary as well as a dynamic function. Faulty co-ordination must be accepted during static strength training.

On the other hand, dynamic strength training has the additional benefit of training one's co-ordination because in this case the muscles are strengthened by movement. Dynamic strengthening exercises can be done using body weight or, as often practised in aerobics, with latex or rubber bands, e.g. dynabands. When doing fitness training one should complete two to six series with 15-20 repeats in about six to eight different exercises (see BOECKH-BEHRENS/ BUSKIES 1995).

Fundamentally the whole body should be strengthened with particular attention being paid to muscles inclined to weakness, i.e. large sections of the back muscles, the stomach muscles, the buttocks muscles and the front thigh muscles (see FREIWALD 1991).

How can I control the amount of strength needed?

Current investigations within the framework of a health-oriented fitness training programme indicate that an individual series of exercises should not be done to a point of exhaustion, i.e. not as far as the maximum number of repeats (no burnout!). Good strength development can be achieved before the muscle is completely exhausted (see BUSKIES a.o. 1994). Also during training, the level of stress can be estimated through the subjective sense of exertion (see Exertion Measurement Scale diagram 2). The exertion felt should be within the medium to intense range, and should definitely not exceed that (see BOECKH-BEHRENS/ BUSKIES 1995).

What achieves good strength capacity?

The effects of strength training rest in an ability of the body structure to handle stress. Thus the bones, for example, become harder and more stable, sections of transverse muscle expand and the composition of the muscle fibres changes. This has a further positive effect on body posture, so that physical problems like backache, spinal difficulties or joint syndromes can be ameliorated or eradicated altogether. In addition to all this, one's figure alters because body proportions are determined more by the muscles than by fat deposits.

1.2.3 Fitness Training Is Flexibility Training

When considering flexibility, we mean the ability to make large swinging movements with one or more limbs. Factors that limit one's ability are the joints and elasticity of muscles, tendons, ligaments and skin. The maximum elasticity is reached between the ages 11-14, after which degeneration sets in quickly without consistent flexibility training.

How can I improve my flexibility?

Flexibility is achieved by stretching exercises, i.e. mainly by exercises in which the muscles are extended. Fundamentally, two methods or techniques achieve this: static stretching and dynamic stretching.

In the area of sports practice, static stretching has established itself as the first technique during which one or more muscles are stretched as far as possible and then held in this position for 15-30 seconds. This sort of stretching should be repeated several times for each muscle.

There are already different kinds of static stretching whereby the methods of continuous stretching and tensing-and-relaxing stretching are recognized (see Chapter 4).

In dynamic stretching, the greatest possible extent of movement by one or more limbs is taken to its limit in two or more directions. During dynamic stretching there should be several repeats. It is suggested that 20 to 30 repeats per sequence should be done in one or two sequences. In recent years this type of stretching has been frowned upon, although it has been proved that this method is impressively effective. When carried out under careful supervision, i.e. avoiding at all costs any jerky and tugging movements, this method can definitely be recommended (see BOECKH-BEHRENS/ BUSKIES 1995; KNEBEL 1994).

When stretching, all the important muscle groups should be included, taking particular care with any potentially weak areas. This means that muscles inclined to contract must especially be stretched. These are the back muscles in the neck and lumbar vertebral areas, the chest muscles, the front hip muscles, the inner hip muscles, the front thigh muscles, the rear thigh muscles and the rear calf muscles (see FREIWALD 1991).

What promotes good flexibility?

Flexibility training promotes considerable positive adaptations of movement and structure as far as one's general health is concerned. The ability of the muscles to stretch is improved by the elasticity of tendons, ligaments and joint capsules. This in turn improves posture and the ability of the body structure to handle stress, and prevents potential problems in these areas, i.e. painful tension in the shoulder area and back.

1.2.4 Fitness Training Is Co-ordination Training

Step aerobics promises to improve co-ordinative skills, by which we mean the interplay of the central nervous and muscular systems. The smoother this interplay is, the more elegant, faster and decisive the performance of the movement seems to be. Under the heading "co-ordination" comes a wide range of aspects that can also be called co-ordinative skills. For example, in this category we include rhythm, balance, agility and reflexive ability (RIEDER/ LEHNERTZ 1991). Innumerable skills such as these are needed during training. The more varied a programme is, the better the chances are of counteracting any deterioration due to aging.

1.2.5 Fitness Training Is Feeling Well in the Here and Now

Step aerobics promises a positive influence on emotional wellbeing, by which enjoyment of life is improved.

Since at least the 70s there has been talk about positively influencing psychological state through sport. At this time American studies documented positive mood changes during and after sports activity and referred to this state in such impressive terms as the "feel better phenomenon" and the "runner's high". By use of these words, a generally improved mood, i.e. euphoric or even trance-like state is referred to, which can be attained through long-term stress activities like running. The researchers were also able to ascertain that feelings of tension and anxiety could be reduced after sport activity.

In Germany, Andrea Abele and Walter Brehm have produced extensive evidence of wellbeing during sporting activity, evidence which is also relevant to step aerobics. From innumerable studies of fitness activity, the authors could prove that one's mood is usually significantly better immediately after than just before sport activity. They investigated running, swimming, aerobics, jazz gymnastics, conditioning, strength training at machines etc. During such exercise, negative mood components are reduced and positive ones are enhanced. Those doing sports feel better motivated, in a better mood and more calm after a fitness activity. At the same time they have the sense of being less tense, less irritable and less lacking in energy and are less depressed than before (see ABELE/ BREHM 1993).

(Aerobic, Fitness with Music, Skiing)

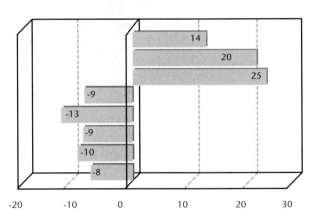

13 courses; N = 240, 3 survey times *=p<0.1 (Abele/Brehm)

Diagram 3: Wellbeing during fitness activities

However, improvements in one's mood do not always take place within the framework of sports activity and are more dependant on various other factors. These factors can affect how the fitness training program is arranged. The following appraisal looks at which factors can positively affect one's mood, under what conditions this happens and what exercise leaders and trainers can practically use in their teaching sessions (see BREHM/ PAHMEIER 1992, BREHM 1995).

Factors	Conditions	Didactic consequences
State of mood	The "starting point of one's mood" influences its alteration. People with a tendency towards bad moods profit more than those in a generally good mood. Awareness of mood is important.	At the start of the lesson, one's attention should be drawn briefly to how one feels.
Stress	One's own sense of exertion must be within the medium range. To exert oneself is no doubt important, but one should not feel overstretched or exhausted.	See to it that the participants neither under- nor overexert themselves. Avoid extreme conditional and co-ordinative demands.
"Rhythmizing"	Sporting activities must set to a rhythm as often as possible. One should also see to it that the training units are continually varied.	Give rhythmic aids e.g. music. Variations of lesson content and incorporation of new and varied exercises.
Switching off/ Relaxing	It must be possible in-between times to lose oneself in the sporting activity without being aware of the surroundings.	Plan to include lesson components, so that the participants concentrate totally on their own body and movement and thus practise helping their concentration.
	Conscious relaxation encourages one's wellbeing.	Insert relaxation exercises.

Factors	Conditions	Didactic consequences
Motives	A motive structure which has proved advantageous is to include those easily fulfilled in the longer term (e.g. getting healthier and more fit, acquiring a good figure) and short-term motives (e.g. exerting oneself).	Make aware of short-term motives, address them and reinforce them with the participants.
Experience/Fun	The programme content must enhance the enjoyment of the experience.	Further positive experience and enjoyment e.g. through communication, a good mood, rhythmic stress.
Contentment	The participants must be satisfied with themselves and their achievement, whereby the assessment of contentment is directed by one's internal body feelings.	Further inner contentment.

1.3 Step Aerobics Programme

A movement programme implies exercise units or lessons based on a clear structure (sequence of movement phases), and well-defined content (specific exercises) which can be repeated at any time.

In order to achieve the aforesaid fitness goals, two programme variations have been set up for step training. On one hand we find programmes aimed at increasing long-term performance potential. In such programmes, usually 45-60 minutes in duration, various step patterns and movement elements follow each other. The aim is usually to methodically work out an established sequence of movements (choreography, combination).

The character of the endurance or choreography phase can be formed in various ways through the expression of movement. At the same time, one can give it a sporting or athletic emphasis, i.e. by repeating many of the steps and only having a minimal co-ordinative section. Dance can also be emphasized, where the choreography requires a high level of co-ordination.

Another differentiation in this programme is based on the type of training. One needs to distinguish between low-, high- or mixed-impact training.

During low-impact training, one foot always remains in contact with the floor. Walking is the preferred form of movement, thus putting only slight load on the muscular and structural systems. This form of training is ideally suited to untrained and inexperienced people.

During high-impact training, both feet briefly leave the floor when running, hopping and jumping. With mixed-impact training, there is constantly alternation between low- and high-impact. Thus the different levels of training intensity are described with concepts of low-, high- and mixed-impact.

The second variant puts its emphasis simultaneously on training long-term endurance potential as well as training strength and agility. This programme generally lasts about 50-60 minutes whereby about 1/3 of the training time is devoted to strength training. Appropriate functional exercises both lying down and sitting up are practised with the step apparatus.

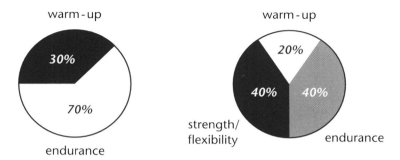

Diagram 4: Evaluation of the lesson emphases

1.4 Step Aerobics and Music

The incorporation of music is an indispensable part of every exercise unit in step aerobics. The motivating and stimulating effect of music has been verified in many surveys. The experience of harmonic interplay between music and movement influences the human psyche. Ideally this enhances wellbeing and mood, creates more joy in performing the movements and increases performance potential. Individuals are constantly warned about the dangers of overexertion and demanding too much of oneself by an upbeat rhythm. Conscientious exercise leaders, trainers and teachers should keep this in mind and see to it that individuals do not trespass their personal limitations (see GROOS/ ROTHMAIER 1991).

In step aerobics, the insertion of music fulfills another role alongside the aspect of emotional experience. Music supports movement in a rhythmic and dynamic way, it steers and harmonizes the flow of movement, and it organizes a chronological sequence of exercises. The styles of music used in the training programmes for step aerobics come in all sorts of shapes and sizes ranging from soul to funk to hip-hop and rock, depending on what suits the participants, making any kind of music viable. What characterizes the music, however, and takes pragmatic aspects into consideration, is the use of pieces that flow into each other (see Chapter 3).

1.5 The Step Apparatus

Using a wooden box as a training apparatus has long since been abandoned by step aerobics, at least commercially. Due to the fact that in recent years many more marketing firms other than Reebok have turned their attention to "Step", there is now a wide range of step apparatus offered from the good-value sort to the very expensive.

Along with the original Reebok-Step, a 15 x 20 x 25 cm height-variable platform covered in a slip-resistant surface, another product from "Forever-Fit-Performance Ltd." in Regensburg called "The Step" has appeared on the market. "The Step" is particularly flexible in its use, as it can be built together in a system of building blocks (see diagram 5).

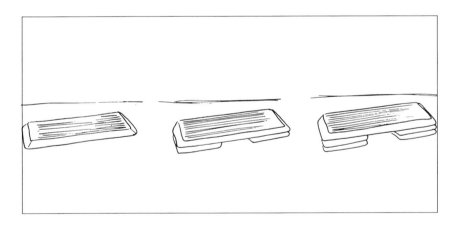

Diagram 5: The step apparatus in a building-block system without supports, with 2 supports, with 4 supports

The various components of the system are made of slip-resistant, elastic, synthetic fibre. The platform (also called the "bench") is 1.10 metres long and 0.40 metres wide. It is 10 cm high and can be altered in its height by putting right-angled supports underneath it. Then, with a support at each end, the platform is raised to 15.5 cm, and with two supports to 20.5 cm. The supports are hollow and thus relatively light.

Alternative apparatus

Exercise leaders in clubs and schoolteachers who want to do step aerobics should acquire permanent step apparatus. However, a step training programme need not be abandoned due to a lack of standardized equipment. We have put together for you a series of ideas and suggestions so that you can teach step aerobics despite missing equipment.

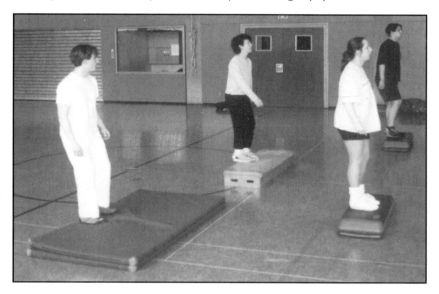

Gymnastic equipment as step apparatus

1. How to turn available gymnastic equipment into step apparatus:

In every gymnasium or sports hall you will find gymnastic mats. Pile these up on top of each other to suit the individual performance level of your participants, ensuring that the mats are not too soft. (Soft floors are inadvisable due to the risk of injury.) These arrangements of mats are so big that at least two participants can train at the same time.

The upper sections of big gymnastic boxes are also suitable as steps, but one disadvantage is that their height cannot be adjusted. In many cases it is advisable from a safety point of view to put thin, anti-slip rubber mats under

27

the box sections. A third possible variant is with jumping boards slotted into each other, which unfortunately is not possible with all makes of the product.

2. Build step apparatus out of wood

Do you remember? Gin Miller developed her original idea on the good old wooden crate. A committed exercise leader from Bavaria sent us the following suggestions for building your own wooden step apparatus.

The step consists of a long, wooden plank (2 cm thick x 30 cm wide x 60 cm long). This plank is screwed into three supports that are each 6 cm thick x 17 cm high. Both of the outer foot supports must be firmly fixed to the upper plank so that the step cannot tip over. The step then also needs a thin rubber underlay so that it cannot slip away on the sports hall floor (safety!).

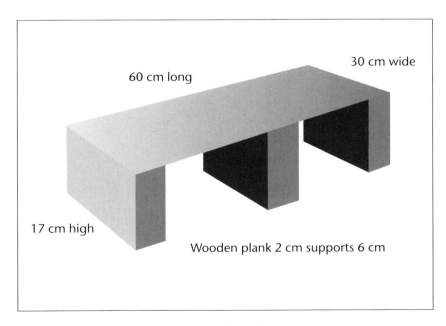

Diagram 6: Step apparatus made out of wood

Any carpenter can make this step apparatus. One could also seek the co-operation of an art or technology teacher at school for building wooden apparatus.

3. Borrow step apparatus from a fitness studio

This admittedly somewhat costly procedure is suitable for clubs wishing to offer demonstrations or test courses in step aerobics. You first need to find a studio willing to co-operate!

2 Step Aerobics: a Trendy Craze or an Established Kind of Fitness Training?

New fitness trends developing from the commercial fitness scene are usually regarded at first with scepticism by experienced trainers, exercise leaders, teachers and academics alike. Although step aerobics has been accompanied by scientific evaluation from American sports scientists, it has not been immune to corresponding scepticism. As with many kinds of sport and fitness activities, many questions about step aerobics remain unanswered. However, some questions are answered in research by the American scientists, Peter and Lorna Francis, together with some research in the German language. Interested readers can study the results of the following investigations.

2.1 Is Step Aerobics an Efficient Form of Endurance Training?

Stamina or endurance is trained when large groups of muscles are moved about over a long period of time. Endurance activities recognized as being healthy are swimming, cycling, cross-country skiing, jogging or running and walking or brisk walking. If one wishes to investigate scientifically whether a certain kind of sport or workout trains endurance potential, certain physiological factors based on sports medicine research need to be studied. As endurance potential addresses the heart and circulatory system as well as the respiratory system, parameters are drawn from both systems for measuring this ability. A classic means of determining endurance potential is to measure the resting heart rate i.e. the maximum heart-beat frequency during physical exertion, the lactate or lactic acid concentration in the blood and the maximum absorption of oxygen. The heart rate indicates the number of heartbeats per minute. The maximum amount of oxygen absorbed (VO_2 max) is the maximum amount of oxygen per minute which large groups of muscles can absorb during difficult intense dynamic work. This classes as a reliable gross criterion for assessing the maximum performance potential of heart, circulation, breathing and metabolism (RHÖTHIG 1993, WEINECK 1990).

In one of the studies commissioned by Reebok, the question was asked whether one could compare the physiological effects from two endurance sports: running and brisk walking. Eight healthy people completed the following tests in an attempt to answer that question: walking on a treadmill at a speed of 4.8 km/hr, walking on a treadmill at a speed of 11.3 km/hr and completion of a step programme on a 25.4 cm high platform to music played at a speed of 120 bpm. The researchers could deduce the following: the consumption of energy, measured over a maximum intake of oxygen, was four times greater when walking than at rest. The consumption of energy when running was three times greater than when walking. During step training, consumption rose slightly by 6% compared with running. Although energy consumption during running and step training were much the same, a declining tendency was noticed for heart rate. So the average heart rate when walking was 163 beats per minute, whereas when step training it was 178 beats per minute, and thus 9% higher (REEBOK MANUAL 1990).

KOBUSCH-NIEDERBÄUMER confirmed this fact in her work of 1994. She carried out an analysis of the physical demands of step aerobics. A control group of 18 people was set up on a bike ergometer and then compared with a control group having completed a step choreography. The results also showed that the heart rate data with equal lactate data were higher in step training than on the bike ergometer. How can we explain this phenomenon? Total body weight is being carried on the bike ergometer, and mainly the leg muscles are doing all the moving. On the other hand, when step training, body weight must be constantly lifted up and down. In addition, there is a continual recurrence of arm movements that are mainly done at chest level or above one's head. In order to supply both arm and shoulder muscles with enough oxygen under these conditions, the blood has to be pumped upwards from the heart. To meet this demand, the heart responds by increasing its frequency.

There is reference to aerobic energy metabolism in training. In healthy people this lies between 2 mmol/l lactate and 4 mmol/l lactate, where "2" determines the aerobic threshold and "4" the anaerobic threshold (see WEINECK 1990).

KOBUSCH-NIEDERBÄUMER shows in her 1994 study that in all the stress areas of low-impact programmes and in 3 out of 4 stress areas of mixed-impact programmes one is dealing with a form of training in the aerobic energy metabolism area. The investigations carried out have shown that step aerobics gives stimuli which are physically demanding but which aim to improve endurance potential. However, exercise leaders should know that it is only a limited kind of control when assessing physical demands only from the heart rate. During intense arm work, principally above chest level, the heart rate readings are above the healthy level, although the physiological demand remains within acceptable limits.

2.2 To What Extent Does the Height of the Step Matter?

Of particular interest is the question to what extent does the height of the step affect energy consumption, i.e. how does it affect the parameters of physical potential? The following tables show the demanding situations, which the participants in a KOBUSCH-NIEDERBÄUMER survey of 1994 had to undergo. They completed a 5 minute step choreography using low- and mixed-impact performance variations. In each performance variation, the step height (15.5 cm and 20.5 cm) and music tempo (120 bpm and 130 bpm) were each manipulated twice, so that the test subjects ran through 4 conditions per performance variation. To establish the endurance potential, both the lactose concentration of the blood and the heart rate was measured at rest and under stress.

Chart 2: Lactose concentration and heart rate depending on step height and music tempo during a given exercise:

	Low-Impact			
	Music tempo 120 bpm		Music tempo 130 bpm	
	lactose (mmol/l)	HR (B/m)	lactose (mmol/l)	HR (B/m)
Step 15.5 cm	2.21	158	2.56	167
height 20.5 cm	2.70	165	2.99	174

Chart 3: Lactose concentration and heart rate depending on step height and music tempo during a given exercise:

| | Mixed-Impact | | | |
| | Music tempo 120 bpm | | Music tempo 130 bpm | |
	lactose (mmol/l)	HR (B/m)	lactose (mmol/l)	HR (B/m)
Step 15.5 cm	3.25	168	3.82	176
height 20.5 cm	3.90	176	4.82	180

The data on the charts shows clearly that physiological stress parameters, lactose and heart rate alter as the step is raised. Now let us look at the low-impact performance. Here the lactose concentration in the blood rises to 2.21 mmol/l when the step is 15.5 cm, and to 2.70 mmol/l when the step is 20.5 cm. In the mixed-impact performance, one can detect a similar increase, where the concentration increases from 3.25 mmol/l (step height 15.5 cm) to 3.90 mmol/l (step height 20.5 cm).

And what about the heart rate? Let us re-examine first of all the data of the low-impact performance. At a height of 20.5 cm, the heart rate increases from a previous 158 beats per minute to 165 beats per minute. In the mixed-impact performance we find a considerably identical increase from 168 to 176 beats per minute. Similar effects are achieved on the step height when the music tempo is accelerated: there is a constant increase in the lactose concentration and the heart rate depending on the step height.

FRANCIS, using a group of young, healthy adults, established this influence of the step height on the amount of energy consumed in a survey at the University of Texas and San Diego in 1992. Stress parameters measured in this case were the maximum heart rate (HR max) and the maximum absorption of oxygen (VO_2 max). The step height is measured in inches (1 inch = 2.5 cm), and you can see very clearly on the following graph that energy consumption rises in direct proportion to raising the step platform.

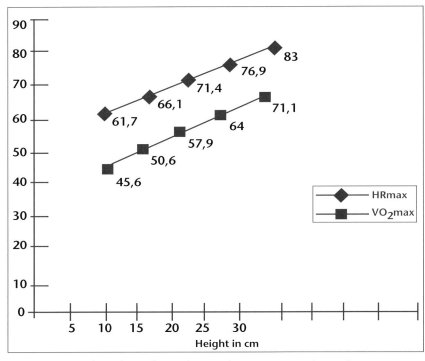

Diagram 7: Alteration of maximum heart rate and maximum oxygen consumption in proportion to the step height

As a result, we can see that the higher the step platform, the more intense the physiological reactions and also the higher the demand on stamina.

2.3 What Effects Do the Performance of a Movement and the Choreography Have?

Let us remind ourselves that the terms low-, mixed- and high-impact refer to the degree of intensity with which a movement is performed (see Chapter 1). Investigations into the physiological effects of certain step patterns can confirm that intensive steps like lunges, travelling steps and propulsions lead to a greater consumption of energy than is the case during a basic step or knee lift step (see descriptions of step movements in Chapters 4.6 and 4.7). It can also be proven that the use of arms affects energy consumption. Step choreographies with arm movements like the biceps curl, for example, cause a 12% increase in the energy used compared with the same choreography where the hands are kept at the waist (FRANCIS 1992).

Yet another increase in stress comes from a particularly intensive type of legwork, that is in the form of mixed- or high-impact performance of steps and step patterns. A survey by KOBUSCH-NIEDERBÄUMER in 1994 confirms this fact. Her test subjects performed the step choreography once in the low-impact variation and once in the mixed-impact variation. The following graphs clarify very well that statistically significant differences exist between both programme variants for the conditional parameters, lactose and heart rate.

Diagram 8: Average group data of lactose comparing low- and mixed-impact

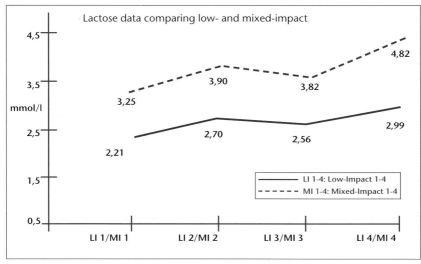

The lactose concentration in the blood and the heart rate after the mixed-impact variation are well above the levels attained after the low-impact variation. The same movement programme during various performance

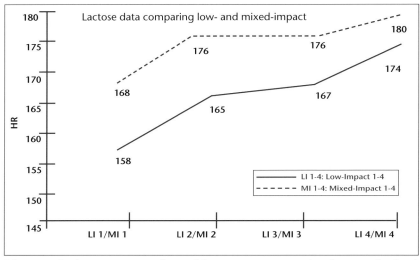

Diagram 9: Average group data of heart rates comparing low- and mixed-impact

conditions (low- versus mixed-impact performance) causes endurance stress of different kinds i.e. physiological demands. A mixed-impact performance makes greater demands on the body.

In many step aerobics lessons hand weights are used. Evidence so far indicates that when using a pound of heavy weights, the subjective demand on the participant or their feeling of intensity alters correspondingly. However, the objective physiological readings showed no change. When heavier weights were used, the participants often complained of shoulder problems. In 1992, FRANCIS concluded that hand-held equipment, even when used properly from a healthy point of view (minimum weight) did not improve the effect of training. He advises the avoidance of hand-held equipment.

2.4 What Effect Does the Music Tempo Have?

An American survey was the first to show the various physiological effects of different speeds of music. The test subjects trained on a 20 cm high platform, and the music changed during the second run of the choreography from 120-128 bpm. The result: energy consumption rose during the second sequence by 4.6% (FRANCIS 1992). Also, as already quoted several times, a survey by KOBUSCH-NIEDERBÄUMER trained the participants with two different speeds. The levels of lactose concentration and heart rate rise when training takes place at a speed of 130 bpm instead of 120 bpm (see Charts 2 and 3). If the music tempo exceeds 130 bpm, there is often loss of movement control. This is confirmed by the subjective experience of many participants. Movements can no longer be performed correctly and there is unavoidably an increased risk of injury.

Exercise leaders should know that the correct levels for a suitable music tempo in a step aerobics lesson should be between 118 and 130 bpm at the most.

From the previous surveys regarding the question of how appropriate step-aerobics is for adequate endurance training we can now draw some conclusions. The demands on the heart and circulatory system can be monitored using three parameters: the height of the step platform, the speed of the music and the varying kinds of movements performed, these being low-, mixed- or high-impact performance.

Exercise leaders should know:
- Mixed-impact performances put higher demands on the performer than low-impact performances.
- Demands increase in proportion to the height of the step and the speed of the music.
- The height of the step and the speed of the music balance each other perfectly: step heights of 15.5 cm coupled with a music speed of 130 bpm create identical stress demands to step heights of 20.5 cm and a music speed of 120 bpm. This comparison is equally applicable to low- and mixed-impact performances.
- Recommendations for training a particular combination of the parameters, step height, music tempo and performance intensity may only be given by considering the performance level and age of participants.
- Untrained and older participants should follow these parameters: low step, slow music tempo and simple choreographies, all done in low-impact performance.

2.5 What Are the Health Risks of Step Training?

This key question applies mainly to the concern that excessive step training could damage the body. There is constant reference to surveys which have proved that runners involved in an extensive training programme have damaged their feet, calves, hips and lower back. The high-impact demands that occur when running claim responsibility for this. High-impact demands also occur in aerobic sports, especially when performing high-impact movements. More recent developments, however, show a pleasing decline of this kind of aerobic exercise.

When considering these results, the constant impact demands when getting off the step platform were seen to be a health hazard. To counteract this criticism in its early stages, Reebok carried out innumerable biomedical investigations in this area. In particular, these are intended to show which forces during the course of step-training have an effect on tendons, ligaments and joints, and which conclusions can be drawn for safe and reliably healthy training.

So that the reader has a brief insight into this area of research, we will now give an example of one of these surveys. The load put on the feet during training can be measured using a biomechanical piece of equipment called a strength plate. This is a metal plate fitted with a highly sensitive measuring device. Not only is the load put on the foot during the upward movement measured, but also the friction between the floor and sole of the foot or shoe.

During the performance of movements, these stresses can be measured 100 times per second and stored in a computer. The following survey should clarify how great the stress load on the foot is during the performance of a typical *basic step* in comparison with stress loads during walking and running.

Eight people separately carry out the following activities ten times:
- Walking along the metal plate at 3 mph
- Running along the metal plate at 7 mph
- Repeated performance of the *"basic step"* at a music speed of 120 bpm on a platform 23 cm high.

We will now outline the stress profile of these three types of activity:

While running, the foot has exactly 180 milliseconds of floor contact, that is less than 1/5 of a second. The heel touches the ground first for about 20 msec. The load put on the foot during upward movement reaches about 3.2 times the body weight of the test subject.

The runner then bounces off the impacts a bit and the load put on the foot during upward movement is reduced by as much as double the person's body weight.

Walking is characterized by two stress peaks. The maximum level occurs 1/10 second after the first floor contact and is about 1 1/4 times the person's body weight. Overall, the foot touches the floor for 6/10 second.

We have also discovered two stress peaks during stepping pace. The maximum amount of load during the highest peak level occurs 1/10 second after the first floor contact. The load then corresponds to 1.75 the person's body weight. The foot touches the ground for 7/10 second.

Now let us compare the three activities:

The load put on the foot during the upward movement of step training is more or less the same as when walking. The first contact with the floor in stepping pace is more of a strain, but considerably less than when running. A comparison of step up with step down shows that steps down generally cause greater strain but can be compared with the demands of walking; whereas steps up show only a slight strain profile compared with walking.

Great care is advised with "propulsion steps", as both feet temporarily leave the ground in this case. When returning to the ground after this movement, the measuring plate recorded a stress load of 2.7 times the person's body weight.

And one final important result: Steps in which one's back is turned on the platform and one descends forward record a much greater stress load than if one descends backward or sideways.

2.6 What Makes Step Aerobics so Attractive?

Alongside the physical effects of training presented so far, all the many positive psychological effects are emphasized again and again in fitness sports.

For the first time a study of the psychological effects of step aerobics training was done at the University of Bayreuth. 103 participants (99 women and 4 men) from 8 fitness studios and ranging in age from 16 to 53 took part in the survey. They were asked about the effects of step training on their general state of wellbeing (see FRIEDRICH 1995/ BREHM 1995).

The results are very clear.

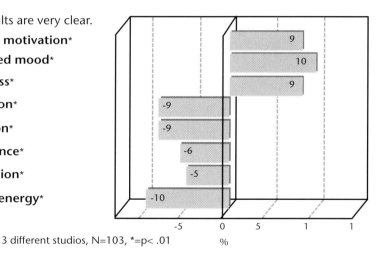

3 different studios, N=103, *=p< .01

Diagram 10: State of wellbeing during step aerobics

The positive contributions to one's wellbeing improve on average by 9-10%. In real terms, this means that the participants feel more active, are in a better mood and are more calm after step training. At the same time, negative influences on one's mood decrease, and there is a clear decline in lack of energy (by 10%) and agitation (by 9%). So the participants feel less weak and excitable after step training, and also less contemplative, depressed and annoyed.

The results fit in well with the surveys on fitness training which show the extent of the difference that step training makes. This speaks well for the strong psychological effect of training.

Alongside these obvious improvements in mood, there are a few other aspects of the attraction to the sport of step aerobics, e.g. the basic movement sequences of step aerobics are skillfully very simple and easily mastered by beginners. By setting them to music and with skilled choreographic work on the part of the exercise leader, trainer and teacher, target groups for training can probably be set up which have otherwise long been regarded with scepticism or rejected altogether. Groups of older people, men, and also young people and school pupils could be considered in this case.

A further advantage of step training is its flexibility; participants of different levels of fitness can train in one and the same group. The step platform with its adjustable height makes this possible.

3   Step Aerobics: It All Depends on the Method!

3.1 Programme Structure and Lesson Concepts

Classical step aerobics lessons structurally follow two different sequences of events. Depending on the emphasis of a particular lesson and the fitness goal aimed at (see Chapter 1), a three- or five-phase structure can be detected. The main lesson emphasis of the three-phase model is obviously to train general dynamic aerobic stamina, whilst the five-phase training lesson addresses both stamina as well as specifically aiming at strength. The following tables survey the content of individual phases, time planning and the right music tempo for each particular phase. The various phases are referred to differently in theory compared with their practice, so we have tried to use the most commonly accepted terms.

The sequences of the 3-phase model comprise:

Warming-up sequence	warm-up
Heart and circulation training	cardiac section
Regeneration phase	cool-down

The sequences of the 5-phase model comprise:

Warming-up phase	warm-up
Heart and circulation training	cardiac section
Recovery phase	walk-down
Muscle training	floor workout
Regeneration phase	cool-down

Time	Contents	Aims	Music tempo	Stress control
45 min 60 min				
15 min 15 min	**Warming-up phase** Partial and whole body movements of low to medium intensity, isolating movement, less complex step patterns and arm movements; "pre-stretch": slight pre-stretching of the muscles.	Preparation of the whole body; stimulating the heart and circulation; psychological preparation for the following stress phases.	128-135 bpm	Pulse/HR, subjective stress sensitivity
20 min 35 min	**1. Stress-phase/Heart and circulation training/cardiac sect.** Step-type stepping patterns combined with various arm movements. Orientation towards: sporting and athletic or co-ordinative dance-like	Improvement of the performance potential under stress of the heart and circulatory system; schooling ones co-ordinative faculties.	118-125 bpm	Pulse/HR, breathing, subjective stress sensitivity
10 min 10 min	**Regeneration phase/cool down** Simple steps, step patterns and movement elements on and in front of the step-apparatus, active relaxation mainly by stretching the muscles inclined to contraction.	Calming the heart and circulatory system; improving mobility; fostering regeneration and relaxation.	< 100 bpm	Pulse/HR, subjective stress sensitivity

Chart 4: Lesson structure in 3 phases

43

Time	Contents	Aims	Music tempo	Stress Control
10 min / 10 min	**Warming-up phase** — Partial and whole body movements of low to medium intensity, isolating movement, less complex step patterns and arm movements; "pre-stretch": slight pre-stretching of the muscles.	Preparation of the whole body; stimulating the heart and circulation, psychological preparation for the following 1st stress-phase.	128-135 bpm	Pulse/ HR, subjective stress sensitivity
10 min / 20 min	**1. Stress-phase/Heart- and circulation training/cardiac section** — Stepping patterns combined with various arm movements. An orientation towards sport-like and athletic or co-ordinative and dance-like movements.	Improvement of the performance potential under stress of the heart and circulatory system; schooling one's co-ordinative faculties.	118-125 bpm	Pulse/ HR, breathing, subjective stress sensitivity
5 min / 5 min	**Recovery phase/walk-down** — Simple steps and step patterns in front of and up and down the step apparatus with minimal stress intensity; stretching, especially the leg muscles.	Calming down the heart and circulatory system; increasing the ability to relax.	120-130 bpm	Pulse/ HR, subjective stress sensitivity
15 min / 20 min	**2. Stress-phase, muscle training, floor workout** — Dynamic stretching exercises especially for the weaker groups of muscles with the step apparatus. (Stomach muscles, shoulder and back muscles, buttocks muscles, chest and arm muscles.)	Improving one's strength potential, especially endurance of the muscles.	100-125 bpm	Pulse/ HR, breathing, subjective stress sensitivity
5 min / 5 min	**Regeneration phase/cool-down** — Active relaxation mainly by stretching the muscles inclined to contraction.	Calming the heart and circulatory system; active regeneration, increasing awareness of the body and the ability to relax.	< 100 bpm	Pulse/ HR, subjective stress sensitivity

(Total Time: 45 min / 60 min)

Chart 5: Lesson Structure in 5 phases

3.2 Structuring Choreographies

Step aerobics is characterized predominantly by step patterns and arm movements able to be set to music in a repeatable sequence both in the cardiac phase as well as sometimes in the warm-up phase. One refers to this in dance terms e.g. movement choreographies or combinations. Depending on the potential, experience of movement and preference of the participants, the cardiac section can range from simple to very complex sequences. In the following chart we have illustrated such a structural ladder:

Choreography	consists of a combination of 4 blocks.
Blocks	consist of two or more elements. E.g. L-pattern +boxing arm and kick-step + clap hands
Elements	consist of a combination of step patterns and arm movement. e.g. L-pattern and boxing arm
Step patterns	are put together from basic forms of movement. e.g. V-step, Turn-step, L-pattern
Steps	are forms of movement e.g. walking on the spot, bouncing, tapping

Diagram 11: Structural ladder of step choreography in the cardiac section

Choreographies are put together from individual blocks. Some authors would use the word "section". Blocks are put together from individual elements which arise out of combinations of step patterns and arm movements. A step pattern contains the basic movement forms: walking, running, hopping, bouncing, jumping and turning in a variety of spatial-temporal and dynamic forms. Steps are in fact what gymnasts call basic forms of movement. Various examples of these individual building blocks are shown in the structural ladder.

Choreographies for step beginners are confined to the building blocks of steps and step patterns as far as the basic elements. Most of the time two to four elements are put together in a sequence of movements (see lesson examples for beginners).

As the participants become increasingly familiar with specific step movements, the choreography becomes more complicated. Step patterns

45

and elements not only become more demanding to perform, also the choreographic structure becomes more complex. When training with advanced participants, it is not uncommon to find eight or more elements combined in two to four blocks (see lesson examples for the advanced).

3.3 Teaching Aspects

3.3.1 Linking Music to Movement

Step aerobics is movement to music. Step patterns and elements of movement are matched to the rhythm of music. The music both structures the movement sequences and determines the tempo of their performance. So, knowledge of the structure of pieces of music and how to use music are part and parcel of the communication of step aerobics.

Basic aspects of music structure

The speed of music is measured in beats per minute or bpm. The beat or time count is marked by the rhythmic percussion instruments. In between two beats comes the offbeat, but in step training, the movement patterns are usually done on the beat. If the movements to the music have a verbal accompaniment, the downbeat and off beat are counted loudly, with the off beat being counted as "and" e.g. "one-and-two-and -three-..."

Melodies as tone sequences of various levels and duration are above the beat. Modern pop music invariably has a particularly clear basic rhythm, in which 8 beats are closely linked together and called a "phrase". The first beat of the phrase is emphasized, and four phrases usually come together constituting a "musical arch".

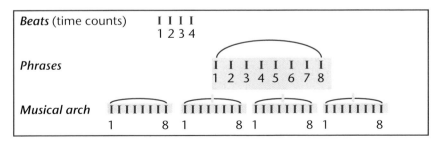

Diagram 12: Basic principles of music structure

Music and movement structure

The structure of movement has some direct consequences for planning choreography.

			Choreography	32 beats or more (max. 128 beats)
		Blocks	8 beats or more (max. 32 beats)	
	Elements	4 beats or more		
Step patterns	4 beats			
Steps	1 beat			

Diagram 13: Structural ladder of choreography and music

Like music structure, choreographies consist of at least one musical arch i.e. 4 phrases (8 beats), or 32 beats altogether. Correspondingly, a movement element or a step pattern consists of at least 4 beats. If the musical structure is used as a base, then one must be in agreement as to how many beats to which a step pattern is performed. For performing a "tap up, tap down" or a "jumping jack" sequence, one needs 2 beats, whereas for a "knee-lift" or a "V-step", 4 beats are needed. This can all be put together in a beginners' choreography as follows:

- *2 V-step*   8 beats
- *4 tap up tap down*   8 beats
- *2 knee-lift step*   8 beats
- *4 Jumping Jack*   8 beats

  32 beats

To put step aerobics across accurately, it is vital to fit the basic steps, step patterns and elements into the basic rhythm. Counting correctly to the music and the introduction, i.e. counting the group into the next movement, is among the most important tools of the trade for exercise leaders, trainers or teachers.

Music and Programme phases

The speed an character of the selected music varies with the individual programme phases (see chart for music speed). However, it is important that the music retains a clear 4/4 rhythm throughout. For the warm-up, we recommend music which encourages movement, but not including jumping or hip movements.

One can increase this in the cardiac section and, depending on the clientèle, the music can then have a driving-on nature. In the subsequnt walk-down, we recommend music which is similar in speed to the warm-up, but should now emphasize the relaxation aspect. A clear structure is vital for floor work. For the cool-down phase, which rounds off the lesson, calm music should be chosen, with the volume turned down, as the music is now intended to form a background for regeneration and relaxation.

A basic guiding principle here is to adapt your choice of music first and faremost to the needs of your participants.

Warm-up phase	*warm-up*	128-135 bpm
Heart & circulation training	*cardio section*	118-125 bpm
Recovery phase	*walk-down*	120-130 bpm
Muscle training	*floorworkout*	100-125 bpm
Regeneration phase	*cool-down*	< 100 bpm

Chart 6: Music speeds

3.3.2 Teaching and Arrangement Methods

As far as the contents are concerned, in the cardiac phase of step aerobics, combinations of steps or step choreographies are taught. The step combinations make this phase interesting. Whilst steps and step patterns are being mastered, the heart and circulatory system is being trained.

At the end of this phase comes a complete step combination which, depending on the level of competence reached by the participants, consists of 2-8 step patterns, which are performed to 32-64 beats.

There are two reasons for careful arrangement: During aerobic endurance training the heart rate must remain constantly raised, which can only be achieved by an uninterrupted flow of movements. In step training, this means that step patterns and movement sequences must constantly flow into each other, also taking care that the participants can reconstruct the various movement elements as planned and also enjoy them, which means learning them well. To do justice to this, two basic guiding principles have been established:

- Outer-form methods
- Inner-form methods

Using outer-form methods, the choreographic sequence is worked out, whereas inner-form methods regulate the repeats of a movement pattern or element.

3.3.2.1 Outer-form Methods

The basic principle here is that the choice of a specific teaching method depends on the aim of the lesson and the target group. For example, to help beginners with their training and to prevent overexertion, the work can be demonstrated without any fixed step combinations. In the "freestyle" method step patterns are repeated but in no fixed order.

During choreographic work, two methods have been established in practice: the "add-on" method and the "link" method, both of which we will explain briefly.

In the "add-on" method each new movement is explained separately and practised before being added to the preceding movements:

- Movement A is introduced
- Movement B is introduced
- Movements A and B are linked
- Movement C is introduced
- Movements A, B, C are linked
- Movement D is introduced
- Movements A, B, C and D are linked

• • • • •

In the "link" method, two movements are introduced and practised at a time; they then form the first link in the chain. After that, two more movements are linked together to make a second link in the chain before they are added to the preceding movements:

- Movement A is introduced
- Movement B is introduced
- Movements A and B are linked
- Movement C is introduced
- Movement D is introduced
- Movements C and D are linked
- Movements A and B, then C and D are linked together

3.3.2.2 Inner-form Methods

When studying inner-form, one must consider how often the elements in the aforesaid sequence are to be repeated. We have chosen a few possibilities for you in the following practical examples.

Method: Block structure

Movement A is repeated 8 times	
Movement B is repeated 8 times	
Movement A is repeated 4 times	8 x (A+B)
Movement B is repeated 4 times	
Movement A is repeated 4 times	4 x (A +B) and
Movement B is repeated 4 times	4 x (A +B)
Movement A is repeated twice	
Movement B is repeated twice	2 x (A +B) and
Movement A is repeated twice	2 x (A +B) and
Movement B is repeated twice	2 x (A +B) and
Movement A is repeated twice	2 x (A +B)
Movement B is repeated twice	
Movement A is repeated twice	
Movement B is repeated twice	

Example:
Knee-lift Step (Movement A)
/ V-step (Movement B)

• Knee-lift step	8 times one after another
• V-step	8 times one after another
• Knee-lift step	4 times one after another
• V-step	4 times one after another
• Knee-lift step	4 times one after another
• V-step	4 times one after another
• Knee-lift step	twice
• V-step	twice
• Knee-lift step	twice
• V-step	twice
• Knee-lift step	twice
• V-step	twice
• Knee-lift step	twice
• V-step	twice

Method: Pyramid Upside-down

Movement A is repeated 8 times
Movement B is repeated 8 times
Movement A is repeated 4 times
Movement B is repeated 4 times
Movement A is repeated twice
Movement B is repeated twice
Movement A is repeated once
Movement B is repeated once
Movement A is repeated once
Movement B is repeated once

8 x (A+B)
4 x (A+B)
2 x (A+B)
1 x (A+B)
1 x (A+B)

Example:

Turn step (Movement A) / up and over (Movement B)

- Turn step   8 times one after another
- Up and over   8 times one after another
- Turn step   4 times one after another
- Up and over   4 times one after another
- Turn step   twice
- Up and over   twice
- Turn step   once
- Up and over   once
- Turn step   once
- Up and over   once

32 beats

Method: Pyramid Structure Variation (Alternative 1)

Movement A is repeated 8 times	8 x (A+B)
Movement B is repeated 8 times	
Movement A is repeated 4 times	4 x (A+B)
Movement B is repeated 4 times	
Movement A is repeated twice	2 x (A+B)
Movement B is repeated twice	1 x (A+B)
Movement A is repeated once	1 x (A+B)
Movement B is repeated once	
Movement A is repeated once	
Movement B is repeated once	
Movement A is repeated 8 times	8 x (A+B)
Movement B is repeated 8 times	
Movement A is repeated 4 times	4 x (A+B)
Movement B is repeated 4 times	
Movement A is repeated twice	2 x (A+B)
Movement B is repeated twice	1 x (A+B)
Movement A is repeated once	1 x (A+B)
Movement B is repeated once	
Movement A is repeated once	
Movement B is repeated once	

Method: Pyramid Structure Variation (Alternative 2)

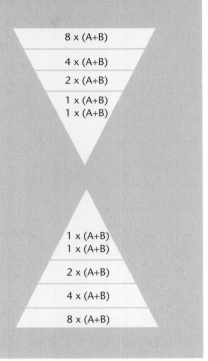

Movement A is repeated 8 times
Movement B is repeated 8 times
Movement A is repeated 4 times
Movement B is repeated 4 times
Movement A is repeated twice
Movement B is repeated twice
Movement A is repeated once
Movement B is repeated once
Movement A is repeated once
Movement B is repeated once
Movement A is repeated once
Movement B is repeated once
Movement A is repeated once
Movement B is repeated once
Movement A is repeated twice
Movement B is repeated twice
Movement A is repeated 4 times
Movement B is repeated 4 times
Movement A is repeated 8 times
Movement B is repeated 8 times

8 x (A+B)

4 x (A+B)

2 x (A+B)

1 x (A+B)
1 x (A+B)

1 x (A+B)
1 x (A+B)

2 x (A+B)

4 x (A+B)

8 x (A+B)

From a didactic point of view, a few aspects should be watched carefully. First of all the individual steps, step patterns and elements are done slowly. Then the tempo is increased and the performance of the movements is adapted to the speed of the music. The principle of adding movements also applies to mastering complex elements. In this case, the movement patterns are worked first and then arm movements are added once the legwork has been mastered. Arm movements and combinations of a more demanding nature are first isolated i.e. learned without leg movements. Only when an individual movement has been grasped are others joined on. This statement fits in with the basic principles of motor learning i. e. from simple to complex, from known to unknown and from easy to difficult.

3.3.2.3 Cueing

An exercise leader, trainer and teacher is as much dependant on his body language as on the spoken word (e.g. counting off) to ensure effective guidance of the learning process of step choreography. This is called "cueing" in specialist circles. Cueing comes from the word "cue" i. e. to give a hint. In step aerobics, this means the verbal and non-verbal aids used by the exercise leader to ensure the smoothness of a workout. Verbal cueing is given loudly with directions and times e.g. "two more V-steps", "another V-step" or "next step to the right".

Non-verbal cueing is both optical and visual where the optical cue uses hand signals and body language; or a visual preview may be given, where the exercise leader demonstrates a complete movement element whilst the participants keep moving and watch.

On the whole, verbal and non-verbal cueing balance each other so that in counting, for example, "4 more, 3 more..." is accompanied by the appropriate hand signals.

The most important of these are shown on the next page.

Apart from these methodically very self-contained methods of arrangement, which come in useful when classical step aerobics training is being carried out, one can also work with open forms depending on the number of lessons. A method particularly suited to use in clubs or schools is working with open-ended assignments, whereby a particular movement exercise is presented, which can then be explored and worked out as the individual participants wish.

For example, in warming up, one could proceed as follows: "Move to music round the step apparatus and find out ways of getting over the step, whilst giving the participants space for developing their own types of movement."

Such exploratory stages can be demonstrated first in schools if one is aiming at choreographies worked out individually. The task could be set out as follows: "Try and join four different types of movement together during a count of 32."

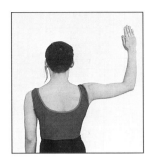

Stop

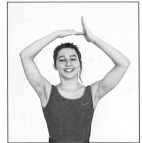

Back to the Beginning

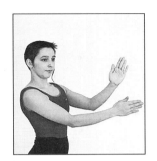

Walk

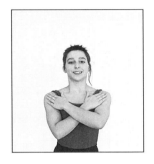

Cross Your Arms

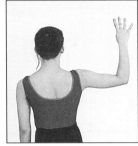

Four More

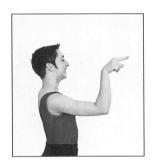

Forward

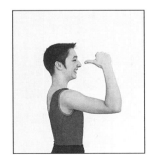

Backward

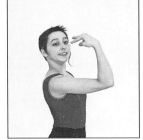

Only Watch

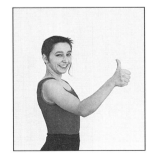

Well Done

55

3.4 Using the Step Apparatus

Setting up the step apparatus in the room

The block position has established itself as the classic way to set up step apparatus during a training session. The steps are set down next to each other with the following row being positioned opposite the gaps.

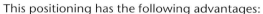

This positioning has the following advantages:
- One can always see the exercise leader
- The participants do not get in each others way
- The participants have definite points of reference
- It is possible to train several people in a small space

Also from a creative point of view a whole range of other positions is possible, as the following diagrams show:

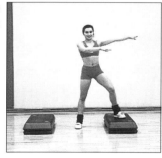

• *Double Step Formation*

Parallel Position

V-formation

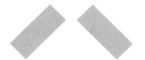

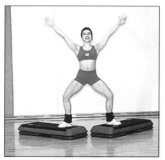

T-formation

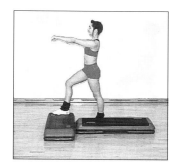

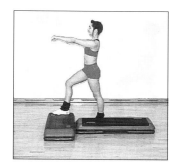

• *Group Formation*

Circle Formation

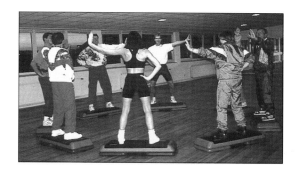

Formation in a Row

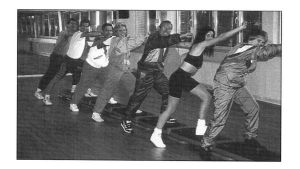

V-formation

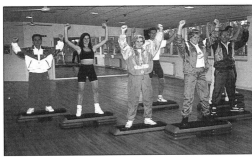

Setting up and using the step apparatus

For step endurance training, the same number of supports is used on both sides of the step within the framework of muscle training i.e. in a floor workout where work is going on with the step apparatus sitting and lying down. This gives the opportunity to set the sides of the step at differing heights so that a slanting platform is available.

Resourceful exercise leaders and trainers can find other interesting types of movement by using the supports or just the platform by itself. You will find a few examples in the following chapters.

Shoes

Step aerobics is done in supportive shoes. On no account should any participants try to train barefoot or with thin gymnastic slippers. The choice of suitable training shoes is an important criterion in minimizing the risk of injury during step aerobics. When buying suitable shoes, one should look for the following features:

- Good shock absorption at the front of the foot
- If necessary, raised heel (to take the load off the achilles tendon)
- Non-slip soles
- Firm lacing to stabilize the foot
- Airy and light, comfortable fit (see also DTB 1994, 11)

4 Techniques of Step Aerobics

4.1 Good Body Posture

Good body posture is important during step training in order to guard against injury. It is possible to consciously work at anatomically and physically good body posture. One should pay attention to following points:
- Legs are placed apart in line with the hips and turned slightly outwards
- Knees are in line with the feet (knee-foot position)
- Legs are always slightly bent so that the pelvis can straighten itself
- Sternum is raised, shoulder blades are pointing backwards and downwards and the neck vertebrae are stretched

4.2 The Correct Step Technique

Good step technique also helps reduce the risk of injury and enhances one's security. How do you recognize good movement practice?

Before starting, ensure that the step apparatus follows safety regulations. Step apparatus with supports must be properly engaged and the platform must not stick out sideways.

Always have a towel on hand for wiping sweat off of the platform. Try to maintain a gap of 20 cm between yourself and the apparatus. The mirror is used to maintain constant eye contact with the platform.

When stepping onto the platform, the foot is placed in the middle using the entire sole of the foot and ensuring that the knee is directly

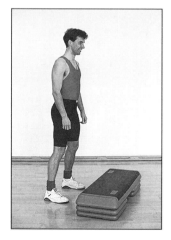

Starting position and correctly positioned step

above the ankle. The whole body is tilted forward in step training with the trunk muscles tightly stretched, and the whole body then leaning forwards from the sole of the foot towards the step.

When stepping off, the ball of the foot is put down first as near to the apparatus as possible, then the heel meets the ground.

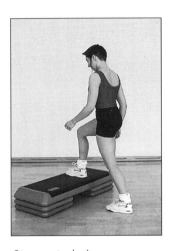 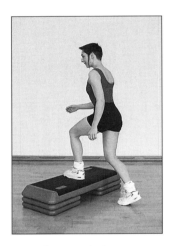

Step up technique   *Step down technique*

4.3 The Most Common Errors

- Never step on or off the back of the step apparatus.
- The balls of the feet and heels should never protrude over the edge.
- Also, during performance of the step movements, the legs must be slightly bent, avoiding bending the moving leg more than 90%. Avoid overstretching the joints, especially the vertebral column. Smaller participants should lower the step if necessary.
- Avoid turning on the leg which is carrying the body weight (see FOX 1991/ REEBOK MANUAL 1990)

Exercise leaders and trainers should constantly draw attention to correct body posture and performance of the movements.

The correct way to lift and carry the step apparatus:
When setting up and taking apart the step apparatus, it should be done in such a way that the back and joints are protected.

The right way to lift and carry

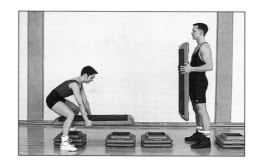

4.4 A Few Key Phrases

Vocabulary Cart. I think this chart can stay the way it is because it helps describe some movements that do not stand out on their own. However, the opening paragraph needs to be rewritten to something like this: What follows is a chart describing the names and performance of step movements.

What does this mean...?	
Step up:	climbing onto the step with one foot
Step down:	climbing down from the step with one foot
Tap:	tipping up the ball of the foot near the stationary leg and then changing over to the moving leg
Touch:	tipping up the ball of the foot away from the stationary leg
Walk/ march:	walking in place
Walk in:	walking parallel in the 1st position
Walk out:	walking parallel in the 2nd position
Plié:	guided bending and stretching of the knee joints
Relevé:	standing on the balls of one's feet
Step touch:	stepping sideways with one foot whilst putting the other foot down to a count of two.
Double side step:	two side steps to a count of four
Grapevine:	sidestep with right, left leg crossed behind right, sidestep with right and tap with left to a count of four
Side to side/ Plié touch:	step outwards from the second position via the Plié into stretching with load on one leg, then changing sides to a count of 4
Hop scotch:	step outwards from the second position, the right and left lower leg are curled round (leg curl)

• • • • •

Squat:	sideways stride to a count of 2
Jumping jack:	jump outwards from the first position and then parallel back with into the first position to a count of 2
180° turn jump:	jump from a striding position through 180°
Lunge back:	from the first parallel position put the right and left leg alternately down backwards and then bring each leg back to the starting position (to a count of 4)
Lunge side:	from the first parallel position put the right and left leg down alternately to the side and then return each one to the stationary leg (count of 4)
Pas de Bourrée:	sideways step to the right with the right foot, sideways step backwards on the balls of the feet to the back right with the left foot, then a side ways step forwards with the right foot to a count of 1 and 2
Repeater:	three or five repeats of a movement within a count of two or three beats.
Propulsion:	increasing the intensity of a movement (e.g. practice jumps step)
Pattern:	step formations
Bridge:	transition from the end of one step to another with 2 steps
Shake the body:	shoulder shaking with the upper body tilted forwards

4.5 Starting and Stationary Positions

Step aerobics has various starting positions that can be used to start step choreographies. The most popular choice of location is from the front of the step. A classic warm-up, for example, is always started in this position

From the front:
Refers to the long side of the step apparatus

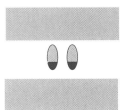

From the side:
Stepping on or off sideways (refers to the left or right shoulder parallel to the step)

From the end:
Starting from the end of the step apparatus

From the top:
From above the step

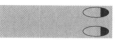

From astride:
Straddling the step

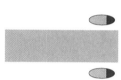

Beside the end:
Sideways to the end of the step apparatus

Standing positions

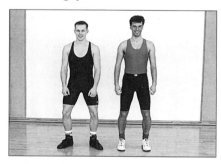
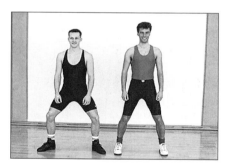

1. Parallel position
1. Outwards position

2. Parallel position
2. Outwards position

The following explanations and lists of basic steps, step patterns and arm movements are, we hope, presented in an intelligible and structured way to the reader. According to our estimations there are already about 250 different step variations that give exercise leaders, trainers and instructors endless scope. The following pages look at the main possibilities, concentrating on step patterns and arm movements that are used most frequently.

4.6 Basic Steps

All step patterns are compiled from the "basic step" and the "alternating step". A complete basic step consists of 4 separate steps that can be performed to a count of 4.

Using the "basic step" as an example this means: step up right (1), step up left (2), step down right (3), and step down left (4). The same leg always starts the movement.

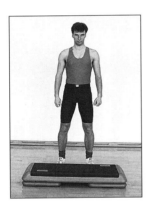
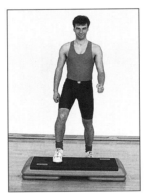
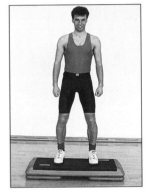
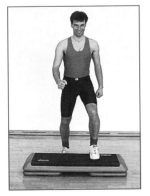
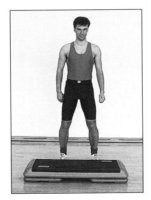

Basic step

For the "alternating step" this means: step up right (1), tap up left (2), step down left (3), step down right (4) or step up right (1), step up left (2), step down right (3), and tap down left (4). The leading leg changes from "tap up" or "tap down" on the counts of 2 or 4.

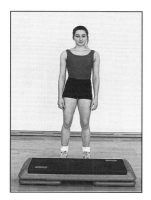 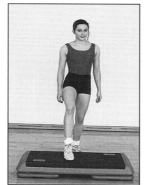 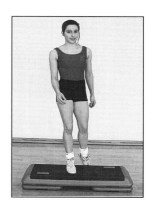

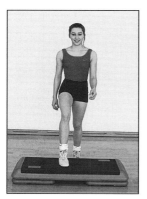 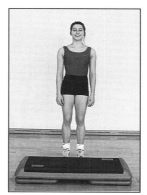

Alternating step

Basically, all other step patterns or variations can be adapted from these steps. Before we describe these variations in detail, we will give a brief description and explanation of the leg movements that have become part of the basic repertoire of aerobics classes. All of these developments can be developed from the "tap".

• • • • •

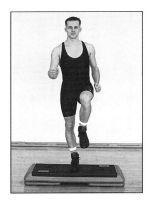 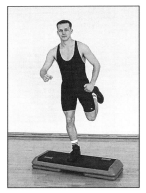 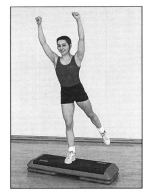

Knee up or knee lift:
Lift the knee to a
maximum of 90° at the
hip joint

Hamstring curl:
Lift the heel towards
one's buttocks

Flying:
Lift up one leg out
backwards. Side-lift
variant: lift one leg out
to the side

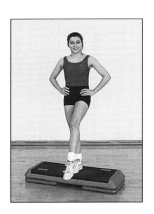 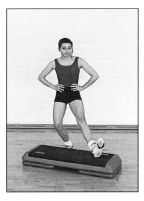

Kick:
Kick the foot out in
front of you

Flex:
Flex the knee and foot
joint resting your heel
on the step platform or
on the ground

66

4.7 Step Pattern Variations

The following step pattern variations are arranged following a simple principle. In the first section we will introduce step patterns that can be done without changing direction. The participant can therefore totally concentrate on performing the step variation without having to bother about the surrounding space. These sorts of step patterns that do not change direction can be begun in a variety of ways. In the second section we will show you how to do step patterns that change direction. Of particular importance are the transition steps with which we conclude in our survey.

Step patterns that do not change direction:

Knee lift step:

Step up right (1), left knee lift (2), step down right (3) and step down left (4), or step up right (1), step up left (2), step down right (3) and left knee lift (4).

Hamstring step:

Step up right (1), left hamstring curl (2), step down left (3) and step down right (4), or step up right (1), step up left (2), step down right (3) and left biceps curl (4).

Flying step:

Step up right (1), fly left (2), step down right (3) and step down left (4), or step up right (1), step up left (2), step down right (3) and fly left (4).

Side-lift step:

Step up right (1), stretch the left leg out sideways (2), step down left (3) and step down right (4).

V-step:

(Step the shape of a "V".) Step up right to the right-hand side (1), change to the left-hand side (2), step down right to the middle (3) and step down left to the middle (4). Change direction with taps to a count of 4.

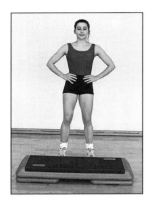 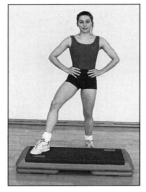 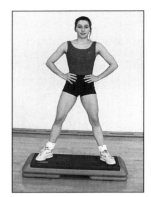

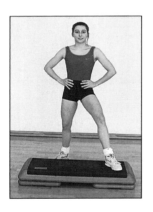 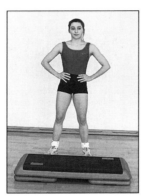

V-step

Charleston step:

Step up right (1), left knee lift (2), step down left (3) and touch back right (4).

Charleston kick step:

Step up right (1), left knee lift kick (2), step down left (3) and touch back right (4).

Straddle up step:

(Start from astride the step.) Step up right (1), step up left (2), step down to the right-hand side (3) and step down to the left-hand side (4).

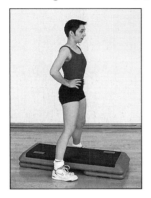 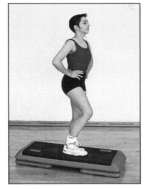 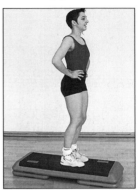

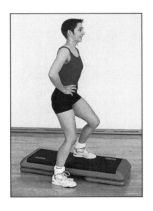 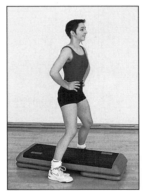

Straddle up

Straddle down steps:

(Start by standing on top of the step.) Step down right (1), step down left (2), step up right (3) and step up left (4).

Up & over:

(Start from the side of the step.) Step up right (1), step up left (2), step down right (3) and tap down left (4).

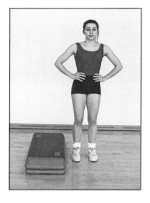 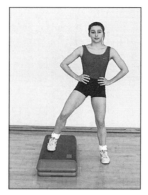 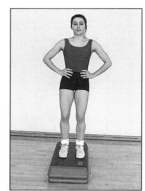

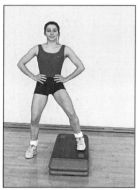 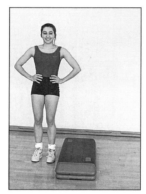

Up & over

Across the top:
(Start next to the end of the step.) Step up right (1), step up left (2), step down right (3) and tap down left (4). (Movement is in one direction across the step, just like "Up & over".)

Corner to corner:
(Start next to the right-hand end of the step.) Complete the same movement as "Across the top" and "Up & over", but diagonally across the step.

Lunge back step:
For a count of 8: step up right (1), step up left (2), tap right backwards (3), right foot back on the platform (4), tap left backwards (5), left foot back on the platform (6), step right down (7), step left down (8).

Pony step:

For a count of 4: step up right (1), step up left (2) and jump over onto the right foot (and 2), step down left (3), step down right and jump over onto the left foot (and 4).

Kick ball change step:

Step up right (1), kick left (2), step down left, right (3) and pause (4).

Step pattern variations that change direction:

Turn step:

(Step the shape of a "U" starting from the right side of the end of the step.) Step up with the right foot in a 1/4 turn (1), step over to the opposite end (2), do a 1/4 turn to the right, step down right (3) and tap down left (4).

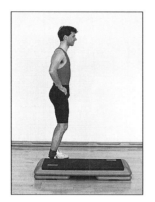
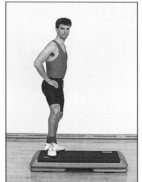
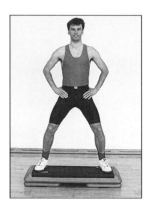

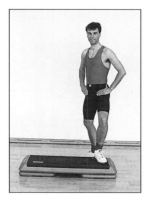
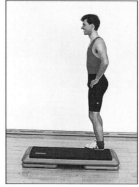

Turn step

Reverse turn step:

Step up right to the left-hand end (1), step up left to the right-hand end, at the same time do a half turn towards the left shoulder (2), step right down to the right-hand end (3) and step left down to the left-hand end (4).

Kick ball change straddle step:

Step up right (1), kick left (2), straddle down left, straddle down right (3) and pause (4).

Piqué jump:

Step up right (1), jump with right leg, bending up the left knee at the same time and turning halfway around towards the right shoulder (2), step down left (3), step down right (4).

Top lunges:

For a count of 8 (starting from the side): step up right (1), step up left parallel (2), striding step to the side and backwards with right foot (3), step up right (4), striding step to the side and backwards with left foot (5), step up left (6), step down right and back with a 1/4 turn to the left hand side (7), step down left (8) (the final position is on the opposite side facing the step apparatus).

Repetition step:

"Flying around the step" is chosen as an example for such a combination of steps. Step up right (1), left knee lift (2), tap down left (3), sidelift left (4), tap down left (5), left knee lift (6), straddle down left (7), straddle down right (8), step up left (9), right knee lift (10), tap down right (11), sidelift right (12), tap down right (13), knee lift up (14), step down right (15), step down left (16), repeat the sequence until the starting position is reached.

Bounce step:

Tap up right to the left end (1), tap up right to the right end (2), bounce with a turn towards the right shoulder.

Transition steps:
L-pattern:

(Start from the front of the step at the left- or right-hand side.) Step up left to the right end (1), tap up right (2), step down right to the right side (3) and tap down left (4).

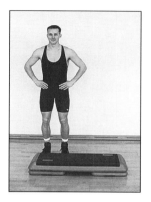
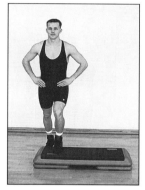
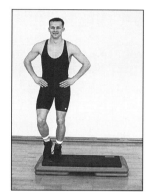
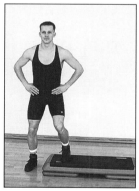
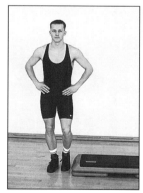

L-Pattern

U-pattern

Step sequence to a count of 8. (Start from the front of the step at the left or right hand end.) To start at the left hand end: step up right (1), tap up left (2), step down and back left (3), step down right (4), step up left (5), tap up right (6), step down and back right (7), step down to the left hand end (8).

73

4.8 Arm Work and Movements

There are various ways of arranging and classifying movements into at least six different categories:

1. Due to the way in which arm movements are performed they may be divided into *groups* as follows: (a) bending and stretching movements, (b) abduction and adduction movements and (c) rotational movements.

2. When using the term *"zone"* or *"level"* we mean the relationship of the body or individual parts of the body to the size of the room. Here we must differentiate between arm movements performed below the shoulders, at shoulder level and above the shoulders.

3. *Directions* in which it is possible to do arm movements are a) above and below, (b) forwards and backwards and (c) sideways and diagonally.

4. By *type* of movement, we mean the skill with which a movement can be performed, which again is defined by concepts such as strength, dynamics and the time factor. Arm movements can therefore be soft and flowing, hard and forceful, strong and fast or slowed down in time. They can be performed on the beat, at half speed or at twice the speed.

5. Arm movements fall into the *"symmetrical"* category if they are performed either symmetrically or asymmetrically.

6. The term *"chronology"* describes the time it takes to perform the movements and differentiates between synchronic and asynchronic patterns.

The categorisation presented here is theoretical. In practice, arm movements can be joined and connected in many different ways depending on the goals of the instructor or choreographic demands.

The following arm movements used frequently in practice are divided into zones, but the description of the arm movements has so far not reached any generally well-accepted term. In the somewhat sparsely available information on the subject, minor variations in the term described can still be found. Some words have been borrowed from the language of dance. This chart can be titled "Vocabulary of Arm Movements". The movements and descriptions can be left as is for the same reason as above.

Arm movements below the shoulders

Clap hands:

At chest height, clap your hands out in front of you.

Walking arms:

An arm movement related to the movement accompanying simple walking.

Biceps curl:

Both lower arms are stretched outwards and upwards, whilst keeping the upper arms alongside the body. One can also alternate to the side and upwards or move the left and right arm alternately.

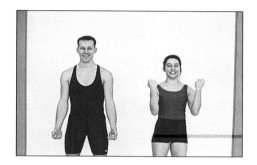

Triceps kick back:

Both fists are placed to left and right of the waist with the elbows of both arms behind the shoulders; from this position, the lower arms are moved backwards and diagonally downwards and bent again. Move the lower arms alternately.

Triceps kick side:

The movement proceeds in the same way as the triceps kick back, but differs in its starting position where the fists are still on the waist but the elbows are held to the side and at a distance from the body, so that the movement runs sideways and down diagonally.

Pumping arms:

Both elbows are held at a distance from the side of the body, whilst the hands are brought one in front of the other at waist height in a jazzhand/fisthand position. From this starting position, push the palms of the hands downwards until the arms are stretched and then bring them back to the starting position.

Pumping arms

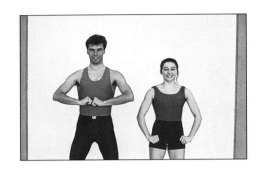

Funky arms:

First, one keeps the upper arms fixed at one's side, whilst the lower arms are raised diagonally 45°. The hands are in the jazzhand position. From this position, the arms are stretched out diagonally to the side and bent as already described.

Criss-cross:

The elbows are held at the sides of the body, whilst the lower arms are crossed at hip level in front of the body. They are then stretched again to the side and downwards diagonally and finally crossed again.

Rolling arms:

The lower arms are turned round each other at stomach level.

Punching arms:

Starting with both hands in the hip position, the arms are alternately punched forwards at hip level.

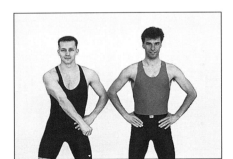
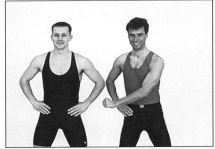

Punching arms

Rowing arms:

The arms, which are stretched out forwards at about hip level, are brought towards the waist by bending the elbows and then returned to the starting position. The movement resembles rowing.

Swinging arms:

The right upper arm is fixed to the side of the body and the right lower arm is placed at a 90° angle in front of the body at stomach level. The left arm is stretched out to the side of the body. The arms fall loosely down to the other side to achieve a pendulum effect.

Deltoid arms:

Both arms are fixed at the side of the body, with the lower arms are held out forwards at 90° angle to the elbow joint. Whilst maintaining this L-formation with the arms, the elbows are brought over the side to shoulder height and then lowered to the starting position.

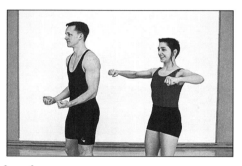

Arm movements at shoulder level

Deltoid arms

Chest press:

The elbows are placed to the sides at shoulder level whilst both fists rest in front of the left or right shoulder from this position. Keeping them at shoulder level, the arms are stretched out forwards and then back again.

Triceps kick side:

The course of this movement has already been described above, but the variation now lies in its performance at a different level, i.e. at shoulder height.

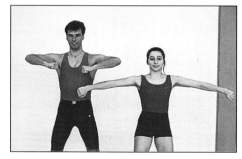

Tricep kick side

77

Butterfly:

The elbows are held out sideways from the shoulders, whilst the lower arms are set up vertically. The lower arms are brought to shoulder level in this L-position back to the starting position.

Shoulder pull:

Both arms are held out-stretched in front of the body at shoulder height. The elbows are then pulled sideways in front of the shoulders whilst the elbow joints are bent at a 90° angle, and finally returned to the stretched position.

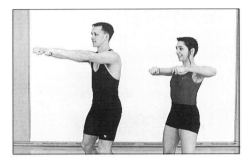

Shoulder pull

Diagonal punch:

Both fists are in front of the shoulders whilst the elbows are to the side of the shoulders. One arm is stretched diagonally across the body, whilst the other is taken across to the side. Both arm movements change sides rhythmically.

Semicircle arm:

One arm at a time (with the hand bent) is brought at shoulder level in a semi-circle in front of the body.

Pendulum arm:

One arm is kept stretched out beside the body, whilst the other arm is positioned only as far as the elbow joint sideways from the shoulder, with the fist of that hand in front of the shoulder. From this position, the lower arms are then swung down to the other side backwards and forwards.

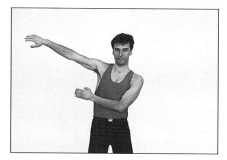
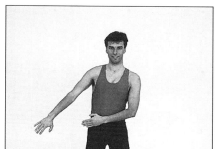
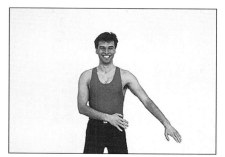
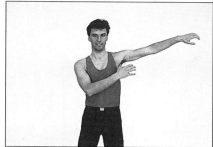

Pendulum arm

Arm movements above the shoulder

Overhead press:

Both fists are positioned at shoulder height near the shoulders, and are then brought closely past the head, stretched upwards and then returned in the starting position. This movement can also be done alternately with each arm.

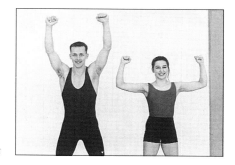

Overhead press

Lateral pulls:

Both arms are held in front of and above the forehead with slightly bent elbow joints. From there, the arms are pulled diagonally downwards guided by the elbows and then pushed up again.

79

Around the head:

One arm is circled round above the head and finally stretched out at shoulder height.

Mixed forms

We now the divide our descriptions into zones of the following arm movements. All of the aforementioned levels are covered during the course of movement sequences.

Lateral raises:

The fists are held together across the stomach, and then, by lightly bending the elbow joints, they are moved upwards over the front and sideways.

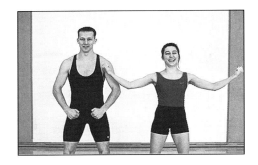

Lateral Raises

Upright rows:

The fists are held together across the stomach, and then, by lightly bending the elbow joints, they are taken in front of the body up to head height.

Circle:

The movement sequence resembles that of "pendulum arms" with the difference that the stretched out arms are taken in a circle down over the side, across to the other side and then high above the head.

4.9 Gymnastic Exercises with the Step Apparatus

The following explanations are intended as a collection of exercises.

Stretching exercises are put into the individual programmes in the warm-up and cool-down. Strengthening exercises are carried out during the floor workout, i.e. the strength and flexibility phase.

Stretching exercises

Calves (Soleus and Gastrocnemius)

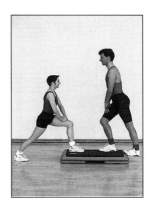

With the right foot standing on the platform, the ball of the left foot is supported on the edge of the step and the heel is lowered towards the floor.

From the first position parallel, the right leg is bent and the left leg put back stretched out in a stride. The left heel is pressed into the floor. Note: the tips of the toe point forwards, the right knee and ankle are above each other and the back is in line with the leg stretched out backwards.

Rear upper thigh (Ischiocrural group)

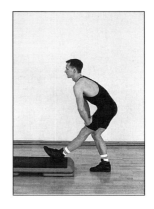

From the Plié position, the weight is transferred onto the right leg, the left leg is stretched out forwards with the ankle bent and the upper body is tilted forward with the back kept straight.

Lying on the back, the right leg is stretched out, the left upper thigh is drawn towards the chest, at the same time keeping the sole of the foot parallel in line with the ceiling.

Front upper thigh (Quadriceps femoris)

From the first position parallel, the left heel is drawn up to one's buttocks. Note: slightly bend the stationary leg, line hips and shoulders parallel towards the front, tense the stomach.

Inner upper thigh (Adductors)

Working towards the outside from the 2nd position, the left knee is brought across the left toes. The stretched-out right leg is pressed into the floor. Lying on the back, the legs, slightly bent at the knee, are pushed outwards.

Hip bender (Illiopsoas)

From the first parallel position, the left lower leg is brought backwards and put on the ground. At the same time, the upper body is supported on the right upper thigh whilst the knee and ankle joints are in vertical line with each other. The left upper thigh is pressed into the floor.

From a stepping position when the legs are bent, the hips are pushed forwards. Note: hips and shoulders should be in line and the back kept straight.

Buttocks and lower back (Glutaeus Maximus and Erector Spinae)

Lying on one's back, the right foot is put down, whilst the left foot is supported on the bent right knee. The arms now pull the right leg towards the upper body.

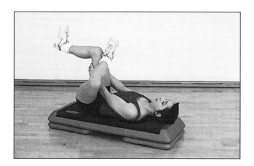

Buttocks/ lower back

Back

The back is rounded towards the outside from a second position with the knees bent and the spinal column upright.

From a sitting position, the upper body is tilted forward, whilst the hands grab hold of the ankles and the back is rounded.

Lying on the step apparatus, both knees are brought up towards the chest and the head is turned towards the knees.

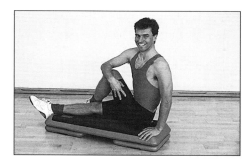

Sitting with legs outstretched, the left leg is crossed over the right leg. The right hand presses the left knee towards the ground, the upper body turns to the left and outwards.

Back muscles

Side trunk muscles (Latissimus)

With the upper body erect, both arms are taken over the head and the right hand wraps itself round the left elbow. The upper body is tilted to the right.

Shoulder blade muscles (Rhomboids)

With the body upright, the right hand rests on the left shoulder and the left hand pulls the right elbow towards the upper body.

Front shoulder muscles and chest muscles (Deltoideus and Pectoralis)

With the body upright, the arms, having been put behind the back, are pushed upwards.

Chest muscles (Pectoralis)

Lying on the back, the bent legs are pulled towards the upper body; both arms are taken behind the head and then rest on the ground.

Side and back neck muscles (Sternocleidomastoideus)

The head is pulled down (double chin position). The right hand clasps the left temple and carefully pulls the head to the right. The left hand pulls against it at the same time to the right and downward.

Neck muscles (Trapezius)

From the double chin position, the head is tilted sideways and the tip of the nose is drawn towards the shoulder.

Back neck muscles (Trapezius)

With the body upright and shoulder blades drawn towards each other, the chin is pushed carefully towards the chest.

Strengthening exercises with the step apparatus

Upper section of the back muscles (Rhomboids)

Starting position: lying on the stomach on the long step, with the knees on the ground, forehead on the step platform and arms bent at the sides.
Doing the exercise: lift both arms to shoulder height at the same time and then lower them again.
Variation: raise the arms to shoulder level forwards and backwards.

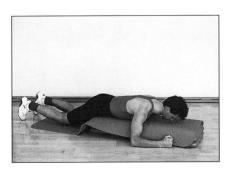 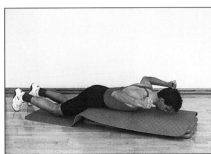

Back muscles

Back muscles (Erector Spinae, Latissimus, Trapezius)

Starting position: lying on the stomach on the long step, with knees on the ground, forehead on the step platform and arms stretched upwards:
Doing the exercise: take the arms over the side towards the back and then return them to the starting position.

Starting position: lying on the stomach on the long step, knees on the ground, forehead on the step platform and arms to the side of one's body with the backs of the hands on the ground.
Doing the exercise: lift head and chest off the platform and turn arms outwards (palms of hands point towards the floor).

All the stretching muscles (Erector Spinae)

Starting position: at the long side of the step with underarms supported on the step, stretch the left arm and the right leg.
Doing the exercise: pull up the left elbow and right knee under the body at the same time, finish with stretching.
Variation: the outstretched extremities are moved up and down with hardly any movement.

Buttocks (Glutaeus Maximus)

Starting position: at the long side of the step, whilst supporting the lower arms on the step; bend the right leg at the knee and ankle 90° (hip joint stretched).
Doing the exercise: lift the leg and then lower it again with hardly any movement.

Rear side of thigh (Ischiocrural muscles)

Starting position: at the long side of the step with the lower arms supported on the step, stretch the right leg.
Doing the exercise: bend the leg at the knee joint and then stretch it.

Inner thigh (Adductors)

Starting position: lie at the side of the step apparatus with the upper leg bent on the step.
Doing the exercise: raise the lower leg from the ground and keep raising and lowering it with gentle movements.

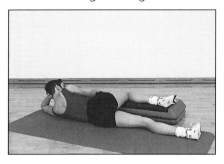 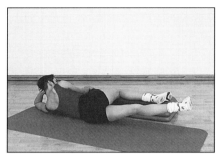

Inner thigh

Outer thigh (Abductors)

Starting position: lie alongside the step apparatus, with the upper leg bent on the step.
Doing the exercise: take the upper leg off the platform and keeping raising and lowering it with gentle movements.

Straight stomach muscles (Rectus Abdominis)

Starting position: lie with both feet on the step platform both hands near the hip-bending muscles on the thighs.
Doing the exercise: roll up the upper body whilst taking the hands past the knees, lower the upper body and return the hands to their starting position.

Starting position: lie with the feet resting on the step platform and keep the hands stretched out to the side near the buttocks.
Doing the exercise: roll up the upper body, turning the arms outward and then lowering them, so that the arms then turn in.
Variation: roll up the upper body, pushing the arms forwards.

Starting position: lie with both feet on the step platform and hands crossed behind the head with the elbows back.
Doing the exercise: roll up the upper body and lower it.

Starting position: lie with both feet on the step platform, with the arms behind the head and hands towards the elbows.
Doing the exercise: roll up the upper body and lower it.

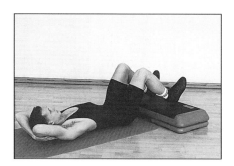 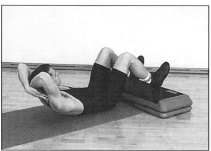

Straight stomach muscles

Starting position: lie with both feet on the step platform, stretch the left arm behind the head and clasp the left elbow with the right arm.
Doing the exercise: roll up the upper body and lower it.

Transverse stomach muscles (Obliquus Externus)

Starting position: lie on the step (which can be set at an angle). Press the heels of both feet firmly into the platform, put your right hand behind your head and then take the left arm diagonally towards the right knee.
Doing the exercise: roll the upper body up diagonally and then lower it.

Starting position: lie on the step. Press the heels of both feet firmly into the platform and put both hands on your temples.
Doing the exercise: roll the upper body up diagonally and then lower it.

87

Starting position: lie on the step. Push the heel of the left foot firmly into the platform and place the right leg on the left knee. Put the right hand behind your head and cross your left hand over your upper body.

Doing the exercise: roll up the upper body, pressing the left hand firmly against the right knee.

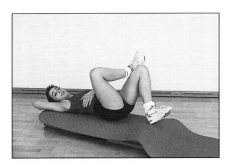 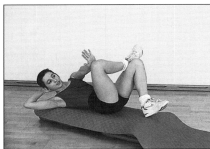

Transverse stomach muscles

Starting position: lie on the step. Push the right foot firmly into the ground and cross the left leg over the right leg. Put the left hand on the left ear, keeping the right arm at the side of the body.

Doing the exercise: roll up the upper body diagonally, whilst the right hand approaches the left knee. Then lower the upper body.

Note with all the exercises: the chin should not be pulled as far as the sternum (double chin position), keep looking at the ceiling. Do not bring the lower vertebral column off the ground, only lift head and shoulder blades.

In starting positions, where the hands are kept behind the head, they actually have a supporting function. Breathe out while rolling up and breathe in when lowering the body.

Chest muscles (Pectoralis)

Starting position: support both hands on the step, stretch the legs out forwards and put the balls of the feet on the ground.

Variation: bend the legs with supporting surface above the kneecap, cross over the lower legs.

Doing the exercise: bend and stretch the arms at the same time (press-ups)

Starting position: lie on the step with the legs bent towards the upper body, arms bent to the side (at shoulder height).

Doing the exercise: arms are bent, with wrists stationary, held out forwards and then brought back to the starting position.

Variation: insert hand weights and "lifelines" or Thera bands.

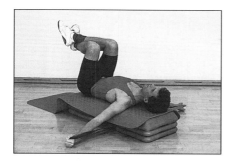 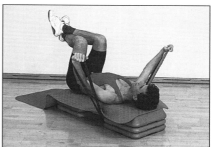

Chest muscles

Arm muscles (Triceps Brachii)

Starting position: sit on the step, soles of the feet placed at a distance from the body, supporting yourself on your hands.

Doing the exercise: lift yourself off the step and, by bending and stretching your arms, raise or lower your body.

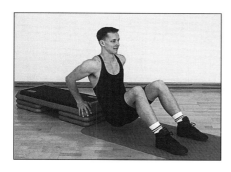 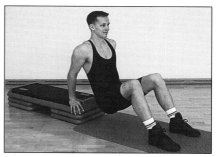

Arm muscles

4.10 Playful Exercise Patterns with the Step Apparatus

1. A different warm-up

The participants go backwards and forwards across the room and move about on the pieces of step apparatus.
When called they
- climb over the step apparatus,
- jump over the apparatus,
- straddle across the apparatus,
- press hard with one leg off the step.

The participants go round and round the step apparatus.
When the music stops everyone
- sits on a step,
- lies on their tummy or back on a step,
- stands on one leg on a step,
- touches the step with an aforesaid part of their body (e.g. elbow, right thumb etc.)

The participants go backwards and forwards round the step apparatus. When the music stops, a number is called out, and that number of people must get on a step without anyone's feet touching the ground.

2. Functional training of a different kind

Alongside the conventional use of step apparatus, the step platform and its supports can be adapted for other sorts of training.

For example the platform can serve as a balancing aid for various functional stretching exercises. We will now describe two possibilities:

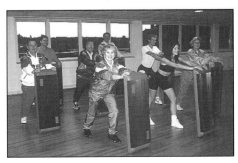

Stretching the calf muscles

Stretching the front upper thigh
muscles

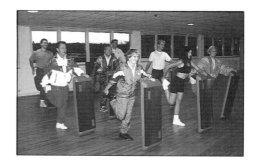

Platform and supports can also be used at weights during the strengthening exercises and here are also a few ideas:

Strengthening the arm muscles
(arm stretcher)

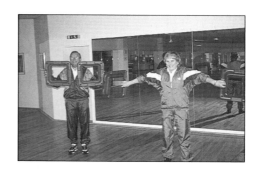

Strengthening the chest muscles

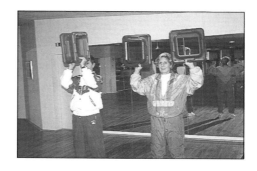

● ● ● ● ●

Strengthening the back muscles/ trunk and leg muscles

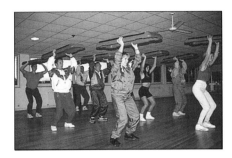 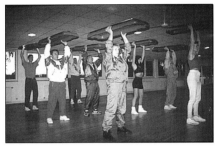

3. Flexibility and co-ordination for the elderly

Using various bits of the step apparatus, and working alone or in pairs, rhythmical movements to music can be done with the supports or the platform. The supports may be moved forwards and backwards, up and down or in a circle.

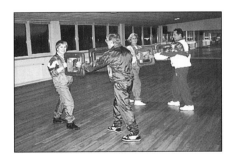

Partner exercises

5 Practical Programmes

Programmes comprise three or five phases as set out already (see Chapter 3). We have now added some concrete examples to each phase, which can be added to training sessions as you wish, depending on the aim of the session, the skill of the participants and the type of target group (building block principle).

5.1 Phase: Warm-up

Example: Warm-up I

Counts	Leg movements	Repeats	Arm movement	Repeats
1-32	walk on the spot	32x	Bring arms from your side up into the air and back again, breathing hard in and out.	4x
1-8	walk out (2. pos. parallel)	8x	walking arms	8x
1-8	walk in (1. pos. parallel)	8x	walking arms	8x
1-4	walk out (2. pos. parallel)	4x	walking arms	4x
1-4	walk in (1. pos. parallel)	4x	walking arms	4x
1-2	walk out (2. pos. parallel)	2x	walking arms	2x
1-2	walk in (1. pos. parallel)	2x	walking arms	2x
1-2	walk out (2. pos. parallel)	2x	walking arms	2x
1-2	walk in (1. pos. parallel)	2x	walking arms	2x
1-32	V-step	8x	pumping arms (1-3) and clap hands (4)	8x
1-32	side lunge (right and left alternately)	8x	no arms	–
1-32	side lunge	8x	triceps kick side	16x
1-16	side lunge	4x	no arms	–
1-16	side lunge	4x	triceps kick side	8x
1-8	side lunge	2x	no arms	–
1-8	side lunge	2x	triceps kick side	4x
1-4	side lunge	1x	no arms	–
1-4	side lunge	1x	triceps kick side	2x
1-4	side lunge	1x	no arms	–
1-4	side lunge	1x	triceps kick side	2x
1-16	side to side	8x	no arms	–
1-16	side to side	8x	chest press	8x
1-16	side to side	8x	no arms	–
1-16	side to side	8x	overhead press	8x

1-8	side to side	4x	chest press	4x
1-8	side to side	4x	overhead press	4x
1-8	side to side	4x	chest press	4x
1-8	side to side	4x	overhead press	4x
1-4	side to side	2x	chest press	2x
1-4	side to side	2x	overhead press	2x
1-4	side to side	2x	chest press	2x
1-4	side to side	2x	overhead press	2x
1-16	side to side	8x	no arms	–
1-16	hop scotch	8x	no arms	–
1-16	hop scotch	8x	punching arms	8x
1-16	hop scotch	8x	lateral raises	8x
1-8	hop scotch	4x	punching arms	4x
1-8	hop scotch	4x	lateral raises	4x
1-8	hop scotch	4x	punching arms	4x
1-8	hop scotch	4x	lateral raises	4x
1-4	hop scotch	2x	punching arms	2x
1-4	hop scotch	2x	lateral raises	2x
1-4	hop scotch	2x	punching arms	2x
1-4	hop scotch	2x	lateral raises	2x
1-8	hop scotch	4x	no arms	–
1-8	side to side	4x	no arms	–
1-8	step touch	4x	no arms	–
1-8	step touch	4x	clap hands	4x
1-32	double side step	8x	no arms	–
1-32	double side step	8x	rowing arms	16x
1-16	double side step	4x	no arms	–
1-16	double side step	4x	rowing arms	8x
1-16	double side step	4x	rowing arms	8x
1-16	step touch	8x	clap hands	8x
1-8	double side step	2x	rowing arms	4x
1-8	step touch	4x	clap hands	4x
1-4	double side step (right)	1x	rowing arms	2x
1-4	step touch	2x	clap hands	2x
1-4	double side step (left)	1x	rowing arms	2x
1-4	step touch	2x	clap hands	2x
1-32	walking on the spot	32x	shake your arms out	32x

94

Example: Warm-up II   right foot leads

Count	Leg movements	Repeats	Arm movement	Repeats
1-16	Plié	8x		
1-16	tip toe (standing on the balls)	8x		
1-8	Plié	4x		
1-8	tip toe	4x		
1-8	Plié	4x		
1-8	tip toe	4x		
1-4	Plié	2x		
1-4	tip toe	2x		
1-4	Plié	2x		
1-4	tip toe	2x		
1-4	Plié	2x		
1-4	tip toe	2x		
1-2	Plié	1x		
1-2	tip toe	1x		
1-2	Plié	1x		
1-2	tip toe	1x		
1-16	bounce	16x	walking arms	
1-16	repeat on the spot	16x	walking arms	
1-4	walk forward	4x		
1-4	walk on the spot	4x		
1-4	walk back	4x		
1-4	walk on the spot	4x		
1-4	walk on the spot	4x	lateral pulls	2x
1-4	walk forward	4x	lateral pulls	2x
1-4	walk on the spot	4x	lateral pulls	2x
1-4	walk back	4x	lateral pulls	2x
1-8	step touch	4x	no arms	–
1-8	step touch	4x	lateral raises	4x
1-8	double side step	2x	no arms	–
1-8	double side step	2x	lateral raises	4x
1-4	double side step (right)	1x	no arms	–
1-4	walk forward	4x	no arms	–
1-4	double side step (left)	1x	no arms	–
1-4	walk back	4x	no arms	–
1-4	double side step (right)	1x	lateral raises	2x
1-4	walk forward	4x	lateral pulls	2x
1-4	double side step (left)	1x	lateral raises	2x
1-4	walk back	4x	lateral pulls	2x

1-16	grapevine step	4x	no arms	–
1-16	grapevine step	4x	shoulder pulls	8x
1-4	grapevine step (right)	1x	shoulder pulls	2x
1-4	walk on the spot	4x	walking arms	4x
1-4	grapevine step (left)	1x	shoulder pulls	2x
1-4	walk on the spot	4x	walking arms	4x
1-4	grapevine step (right)	1x	shoulder pulls	2x
1-4	side lunge (left/ right)	2x	diagonal punch	2x
1-4	grapevine step (left)	1x	shoulder pulls	2x
1-4	side lunge (left/ right)	2x	diagonal punch	2x
1-4	grapevine step (right) - to a count of 4, tap on the right end of the step.	1x	punching arms (1-3) - to a count of 4 clap hands	3x - 1x
1-4	grapevine step (left) - to a count of 4, tap on the left end of the step.	1x	punching arms (1-3) - to a count of 4 clap hands	3x - 1x
1-4	grapevine step (right) - to a count of 4, tap on the right end of the step.	1x	punching arms (1-3) - to a count of 4 clap hands	3x - 1x
1-4	grapevine step (left) - to a count of 4, tap on the left end of the step.	1x	punching arms (1-3) - to a count of 4 clap hands	3x - 1x
1-4	grapevine step (right) - to a count of 4, tap on the right end of the step.	1x	circle arms (1-3) - d. clap (4)	1x - 2x
1-4	grapevine step (left) - to a count of 4, tap on the left end of the step.	1x	circle arms (1-3) - d. clap (4)	1x - 2x
1-4	grapevine with doubletap	1x	circle arms (1-3) - d. clap (4)	1x - 2x
1-4	grapevine with doubletap	1x	circle arms (1-3) - d. clap (4)	1x - 2x
1-32	grapevine step	8x	circle arms with clap hands on a count of 4	8x
1-32	double side step	8x	pendulum arms	8x
1-32	step touch	16x	clap hands	16x
1-32	walk on the spot 32x	32x	alternately circling the arms up and down (to a count of 8)	4x
1-16	bounce	16x	shake the arms out loosely	16x
1-16	Plié (1 pos. parallel)	8x	keep your hands on your waist	–

5.2 Phase: Pre-stretch

Example: Pre-stretch

Starting position: on the top

Muscles used	Description of exercise
Calf (right)	The left foot is on the platform, the ball of the right foot is supported on the edge of the step, and the heel is pressed towards the ground
Rear thigh muscles (left)	The right foot is placed in front of the step apparatus, the left heel is supported on the platform with leg outstretched. The right leg is bent at the knee, whilst the buttocks are pushed back and the upper body tilted forward to compensate. The arms are brought from the side to the front.
Front thigh muscles (left)	The upper body is rolled up with the left heel parallel to the buttocks. The right knee is then bent, buttocks tensed and stomach pulled in. The right arm is raised.
Hip bender (left)	The right leg is bent at the knee and the left leg stretched out backwards. The upper body is thus supported on the right thigh and the arms are placed on the platform. The left leg is taken back parallel into the first position, and the upper body rolled up.
Back muscles	Both legs are bent (Plié), the upper body is tilted forwards keeping the back straight whilst at the same time the hands are clasped behind the thighs. The back is rounded from this position. Roll up to a standing position.
Side body muscles (left)	Whilst standing upright, both arms are raised above the head and the right/ left hand clasps the right/ left elbow. The upper body is tilted sideways.

Starting position: on the top

The stretching exercises are finally done in the same order but on the other side.

5.3 Phase: Cardio Section/Choreography

Examples of ten different choreographies are given. For six of them there are explicit instructions.

| Target group | Emphasis | | | |
	sporting/athletic		dance-like/ co-ordinative	
Beginners	1	2	3	4
Advanced	5	6	7	8
Experts	9		10	

1-10: Number of the choreography

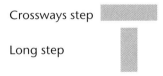

Crossways step

Long step

Diagram 14: An overview of the step choreographies

Choreography 1

Sporting/athletic beginners

Counts	Leg movements	Repeats	Arm movement	Repeats
1-8	hamstring curl	2x	biceps curl	4x
9-16	knee lift step	2x	overhead press	4x
17-24	hamstring curl	2x	biceps curl	4x
25-32	knee lift step	2x	overhead press	4x

Choreographic instruction:

Counts	Leg movement	Repeats	Arm movement	Repeats
1-32	basic step (right foot leads)	8x	hands on waist	
1-16	walking on the spot with tap left to a count of 16	16x	hands on waist	
1-32	basic step (left foot leads)	8x	hands on waist	
1-16	walking on the spot with tap right to a count of 16	16x	hands on waist	
1-32	alternating tap with tap to a count of 2	8x	hands on waist	
1-32	hamstring curl	8x	hands on waist	
1-32	hamstring curl	8x	biceps curl	16x
1-16	hamstring curl	4x	hands on waist	
1-16	hamstring curl	4x	biceps curl	8x
1-8	hamstring curl	2x	hands on waist	
1-8	hamstring curl	2x	biceps curl	4x
1-32	alternating tap with tap to a count of 2	8x		
1-32	knee lift step	8x	hands on waist	
1-32	knee lift step	8x	overhead press	16x
1-16	knee lift step	4x	hands on waist	
1-16	knee lift step	4x	overhead press	8x
1-8	knee lift step	2x	hands on waist	
1-8	knee lift step	2x	overhead press	4x
1-32	hamstring curl	8x	hands on waist	
1-32	hamstring curl	8x	biceps curl	16x
1-32	knee lift step	8x	hands on waist	
1-32	knee lift step	8x	overhead press	16x
1-16	hamstring curl	4x	hands on waist	
1-16	hamstring curl	4x	biceps curl	8x
1-16	knee lift step	4x	hands on waist	
1-16	knee lift step	4x	overhead press	8x
1-8	hamstring curl	2x	hands on waist	
1-8	hamstring curl	2x	biceps curl	4x
1-8	knee lift step	2x	hands on waist	
1-8	knee lift step	2x	overhead press	4x
1-8	hamstring curl	2x	hands on waist	
1-8	hamstring curl	2x	biceps curl	4x
1-8	knee lift step	2x	hands on waist	
1-8	knee lift step	2x	overhead press	4x

Choreography 2

Sporting/athletic beginners

Counts	Leg movements	Repeats	Arm movement	Repeats
1-8	V-step	2x	chest press	
9-16	turn step	2x	butterfly	
17-24	V-step	2x	chest press	
25-32	turn step	2x	butterfly	

Choreographic instruction

Counts	Leg movements	Repeats	Arm movement	Repeats
1-32	basic steps (right foot leads)	8x	hands on waist	
1-16	walking on the spot with tap left to a count of 16	16x	hands on waist	
1-32	basic step (left foot leads)	8x	hands on waist	
1-16	walking on the spot with tap right to a count of 16	16x	hands on waist	
1-32	alternating step with tap to a count of 4	8x	hands on waist	
1-32	V-step	8x	hands on waist	
1-32	V-step	8x	chest press	16x
1-16	V-step	4x	hands on waist	
1-16	V-step	4x	chest press	8x
1-8	V-step	2x	hands on waist	
1-8	V-step	2x	chest press	4x
1-8	V-step	2x	hands on waist	
1-8	V-step	2x	chest press	4x
over 1-8 back to 1-32				
1-32	alternating step right with tap to a count of 4	8x	hands on waist	
1-32	U-step	8x	hands on waist	
1-32	turn step	8x	hands on waist	
1-16	U-step	4x	hands on waist	
1-16	U-step	4x	butterfly	8x
1-8	U-step	2x	hands on waist	
1-8	U-step	2x	butterfly	4x
1-32	turn step	8x	hands on waist	
1-32	turn step	8x	butterfly	16x
1-16	turn step	4x	hands on waist	
1-16	turn step	4x	butterfly	8x

1-8	turn step	2x	hands on waist	
1-8	turn step	2x	butterfly	4x
1-32	U-step	8x	hands on waist	
1-16	V-step	4x	hands on waist	
1-16	V-step	4x	chest press	
1-8	V-step	2x	hands on waist	
1-8	V-step	2x	chest press	
1-16	turn step	4x	hands on waist	
1-16	turn step	4x	butterfly	
1-8	turn step	2x	hands on waist	
1-8	turn step	2x	butterfly	
1-16	V-step	4x	chest press	
1-16	turn step	4x	butterfly	
1-8	V-step	2x	chest press	
1-8	turn step	2x	butterfly	
1-8	V-step	2x	chest press	
1-8	turn step	2x	butterfly	

Can be repeated if desired.

Choreography 3

Target group: beginners/emphasis: dancing/co-ordinative
(Note: unless otherwise instructed, start with the right foot)

Counts	Leg movements	Rpts.	Arm movement	Rpts.
1-8	knee lift step alternately to the left or right diagonally	2x	1, 2: circling both arms with jazzhands; 3, 4: pumping arms	2x
9-16	side lift step alternately to the left or right diagonally	2x	criss-cross arms with 2 finger snaps	2x
17-24	knee lift step alternately to the left or right diagonally	2x	1, 2: circling both arms with jazzhands; 3, 4: pumping arms	2x
25-32	side lift step alternately to the left or right diagonally	2x	criss-cross arms with 2 finger snaps	2x

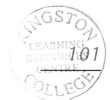

Choreographic instruction

Counts	Leg movements	Rpts.	Arm movement	Rpts.
1-32	alternating step with tap to a count of 2 to the front	8x	hands on waist	
1-32	knee lift step	8x	hands on waist	
1-32	knee lift step	8x	1, 2: circling both arms with jazzhands; 3, 4: pumping arms	8x
1-32	knee lift step	8x	hands on waist	
1-32	knee lift step	8x	1, 2: circling both arms with jazzhands; 3, 4: pumping arms	8x
1-16	knee lift step	4x	hands on waist	
1-16	knee lift step	4x	1, 2: circling both arms with jazzhands; 3, 4: pumping arms	4x
1-16	knee lift step	4x	hands on waist	
1-16	knee lift step	4x	1, 2: circling both arms with jazzhands; 3, 4: pumping arms	4x
1-8	knee lift step	2x	hands on waist	
1-8	knee lift step	2x	1, 2: circling both arms with jazzhands; 3, 4: pumping arms	2x
1-8	knee lift step	2x	hands on waist	
1-8	knee lift step	2x	1, 2: circling both arms with jazzhands; 3, 4: pumping arms	2x
1-32	alternating step with tap to a count of 2	8x	hands on waist	
1-32	side lift step	8x	hands on waist	
1-32	side lift step	8x	criss-cross arms with snaps on 2	8x
1-32	side lift step	8x	hands on waist	
1-32	side lift step	8x	criss-cross arms with snaps on 2	8x
1-16	side lift step	4x	hands on waist	
1-16	side lift step	4x	criss-cross arms with snaps on 2	4x
1-16	side lift step	4x	hands on waist	
1-16	side lift step	4x	criss-cross arms with snaps on 2	4x
1-8	side lift step	2x	hands on waist	
1-8	side lift step	2x	criss-cross arms with snaps on 2	2x
1-8	side lift step	2x	hands on waist	
1-8	side lift step	2x	criss-cross arms with snaps on 2	2x
1-32	alternating step with tap to a count of 2 to the front	8x	hands on waist	
1-32	alternating step with tap to a count of 2 diagonally	8x	hands on waist	

1-32	knee lift step alternately to the left and right diagonally	8x	hands on waist	
1-32	knee lift step alternately to the left and right diagonally	8x	1, 2: circling both arms with jazzhands; 3, 4: pumping arms	8x
1-16	knee lift step alternately to the left and right diagonally	4x	hands on waist	
1-16	knee lift step alternately to the left and right diagonally	4x	1, 2: circling both arms with jazzhands; 3, 4: pumping arms	4x
1-8	knee lift step alternately to the left and right diagonally	2x	hands on waist	
1-8	knee lift step alternately to the left and right diagonally	2x	1, 2: circling both arms with jazzhands; 3, 4: pumping arms	2x
1-8	knee lift step alternately to the left and right diagonally	2x	hands on waist	
1-8	knee lift step alternately to the left and right diagonally	2x	1, 2: circling both arms with jazzhands; 3, 4: pumping arms	2x
1-32	side lift step alternately to the left and right diagonally	8x	hands on waist	8x
1-32	side lift step alternately to the left and right diagonally	8x	criss-cross arms with snaps on 2	8x
1-16	side lift step alternately to the left and right diagonally	4x	hands on waist	4x
1-16	side lift step alternately to the left and right diagonally	4x	criss-cross arms with snaps on 2	4x
1-8	side lift step alternately to the left and right diagonally	2x	hands on waist	2x
1-8	side lift step alternately to the left and right diagonally	2x	criss-cross arms with snaps on 2	2x
1-8	side lift step alternately to the left and right diagonally	2x	hands on waist	2x
1-8	side lift step alternately to the left and right diagonally	2x	criss-cross arms with snaps on 2	2x
1-32	knee lift step alternately to the left and right diagonally	8x	1, 2: circling both arms with jazzhands; 3, 4: pumping arms	8x
1-32	side lift step alternately to the left and right diagonally	8x	criss-cross arms with snaps on 2	8x
1-16	knee lift step alternately to the left and right diagonally	4x	1, 2: circling both arms with jazzhands; 3, 4: pumping arms	4x
1-16	side lift step alternately to the left and right diagonally	4x	criss-cross arms with snaps on 2	4x

1-8	knee lift step alternately to the left and right diagonally	2x	1, 2: circling both arms with jazzhands; 3, 4: pumping arms	2x
1-8	side lift step alternately to the left and right diagonally	2x	criss-cross arms with snaps on 2	2x
1-8	knee lift step alternately to the left and right diagonally	2x	1, 2: circling both arms with jazzhands; 3, 4: pumping arms	2x
1-8	side lift step alternately to the left and right diagonally	2x	criss-cross arms with snaps on 2	2x

Choreography 4

Target group: Beginners – emphasis: dancing/co-ordinative
Note: unless otherwise instructed, start with the right foot

Counts	Leg movements	Repeats	Arm movement	Repeats
1-4			right arm "around the head"	1x
5-8	turn step left	1x	circle arms	1x
9-12	turn step right	1x	right arm "around the head"	1x
13-16	turn step left	1x	circle arms	1x
verbal instruction during "up & over right": immediately add an "up & over left"				
17-20	turn step left	1x	circle arms	1x
21-24	turn step right	1x	right arm "around the head"	1x
25-28	turn step right	1x	circle arms	1x
29-32	turn step left	1x	left arm "around the head"	1x

Choreographic Instruction

Counts	Leg movements	Rpts.	Arm movement	Rpts.
1-32	alternating step with tap to a count of 4 to the front	8x	hands on waist	
1-32	U-step to the front	8x	hands on waist	
1-32	turn step	8x	hands on waist	
1-32	U-step to the front	8x	hands on waist	
1-32	alternating step	8x	hands on waist	
1-32	alternating step	8x	right and left arm alternately: "around the head"	8x
1-32	U-step to the front	8x	right and left arm alternately: "around the head"	8x
1-32	turn step	8x	right and left arm alternately: "around the head"	8x
1-16	turn step	4x	hands on waist	

1-16	turn step	4x	right and left arm alternately: "around the head"	4x
1-8	turn step	2x	hands on waist	
1-8	turn step	2x	right and left arm alternately: "around the head"	2x
1-8	turn step	2x	hands on waist	
1-8	turn step	2x	right and left arm alternately: "around the head"	2x
1-32	up tap, down tap (standing to the side), right foot leads	8x	hands on waist	
1-28	up & over (= double side step)/ to the right	7x	hands on waist	
29-32	is an up tap down tap (left foot leads)	1x	hands on waist	
1-28	up tap down tap	7x	hands on waist	
29-32	up & over (to the left)	1x	hands on waist	
1-32	up & over	8x	circle arms	8x
1-16	up & over	4x	hands on waist	4x
1-16	up & over	4x	circle arms	4x
1-8	up & over	2x	hands on waist	2x
1-8	up & over	2x	circle arms	2x
1-8	up & over	2x	hands on waist	2x
1-8	up & over	2x	circle arms	2x
1-32	turn step	8x	right and left arm alternately: "around the head"	8x
1-32	up & over	8x	circle arms	8x
1-16	turn step	4x	right and left arm alternately: "around the head"	4x
1-16	up & over	4x	circle arms	4x
1-8	turn step	2x	right and left arm alternately: "around the head"	2x
1-8	up & over	2x	circle arms	2x
1-4	turn step	1x	hands on waist	
1-12	up tap down tap (left}	3x	hands on waist	
1-32	up & over (verbal cueing – announce next sequence)	8x	hands on waist	
1-4	turn step left	1x	left arm "around the head"	1x
5-8	up & over right	1x	circle arms	1x
9-12	turn step left	1x	right arm "around the head"	1x
13-16	up & over right	1x	circle arms	1x

105

verbal instruction during up and over right: immediately add an "up and over left"				
17-20	up & over left	1x	circle arms	1x
21-24	turn step right	1x	right arm "around the head"	1x
25-28	up & over right	1x	circle arms	1x
29-32	turn step left	1x	left arm "around the head"	1x

Choreography 5

Target group: Advanced –
Emphasis: combination (sporting-athletic) Crossways step

Elements	Cnts.	Pos. at the step	Leg movements	Rpts.	Arm movements	Rpts.
Element A	1-8		lunge back step	1x	triceps kick back (during both lunges)	2x
	1-8		lunge side step	1x	diagonal punch (during both lunges)	2x
	1-8		lunge back step	1x	triceps kick back	2x
	1-8		lunge side step	1x	diagonal punch	2x
Element B	1-16		U-pattern as a variation; i.e. instead of up tap down tap, up knee-lift, touch, side-lift, touch, knee-lift down, down tap and likewise to the other side.	2x	alternately shoulder pull and deltoid arms	4x 4x
Element C	1-32		fly around the step	1x	walking arms	32x
Element D	1-32		V-step (alternately right and left)	8x	chest press	16x

Choreography 6

Target group: Advanced – Emphasis: sporting-athletic – Long step

Elements	Cnts.	Leg movements	Rpts.	Arm movements	Rpts.
		Starting position: on the top			
Element A	1-32	walk on the top	32x		
	1-32	walk on the top with tap to a count of 4 (starting on the right foot)	8x		
	1-32	alternately straddle down, down up tap (starting on the right foot)= alternately straddle	8x		
	1-32	straddle down, down up tap (starting on the right foot) on the eight repeat, tap to a count of 4, so that you change sides.	8x	or alternatively straddle down (right leads) alternating straddle	7x
	1-32	straddle down, down up tap (starting on the left foot) on the eight repeat, tap to a count of 4, so that you change sides.	8x	straddle down (left leads) alternating straddle	1x 7x
	1-16	straddle down right alternating straddle	3x 1x		1x
	1-16	straddle down left alternating straddle	3x 1x		
	1-8	straddle down right alternating straddle	1x 1x		
	1-8	straddle down left alternating straddle	1x 1x		
	1-8	straddle down right alternating straddle	1x 1x		
	1-8	straddle down left alternating straddle	1x 1x		
	1-32	alternating straddle	8x		
	1-32	alternating straddle	8x	alternately: 1,2: overhead press; 3, 4: chest press	8x
	1-16	alternating straddle	4x	alternately: 1,2: overhead press; 3, 4: chest press	4x
	1-16	alternating straddle	4x		
Element B	1-32	walk on the top	32x		
	1-32	side centre right, side centre left on the top	8x		

107

	1-32	side centre right, left diagonally = side lunge alternately	16x		
	1-32	side centre left, to the right diagonally	16x		
	1-32	side lunge alternately (starting on the r. foot)	16x	diagonal punch	16x
	1-16	side lunge alternately right and left	4x		
	1-16	side lunge alternately right and left	4x	diagonal punch	8x
Element A+B	1-32	walk on the top	32x		
	1-16	straddle down right alternating straddle	3x 1x		
	1-16	straddle down left alternating straddle	3x 1x	alternately: 1,2: overhead press; 3, 4: chest press	4x
	1-16	side lunge alternately right and left (starting on the right foot)	4x		
	1-16	side lunge alternately right and left (starting on the right foot)	4x	diagonal punch	8x
	1-16	straddle down right alternating straddle	3x 1x	alternately: 1,2: overhead press; 3, 4: chest press	4x
	1-16	straddle down left alternating straddle	3x 1x	alternately: 1,2: overhead press; 3, 4: chest press	4x
	1-32	side lunge alternately right and left (starting on the right foot)	8x	diagonal punch	16x
	1-8	straddle down right alternating straddle	1x 1x	alternately: 1,2: overhead press; 3, 4: chest press	2x
	1-8	straddle down left alternating straddle	1x 1x	alternately: 1,2: overhead press; 3, 4: chest press	2x
	1-16	side lunge alternately right and left (starting on the right foot)	4x	diagonal punch	8x
Element C	1-32	walk on the top	32x		
	1-32	lunge back alternately right and left (starting on the right foot)	8x		

	1-32	lunge back alternately right and left (starting on the right foot)	8x	rowing arms	16x
	1-16	lunge back alternately right and left (starting on the right foot)	4x	no arms	–
	1-16	lunge back alternately right and left (starting on the right foot)	4x	rowing arms	8x
Element A+B+C	1-32	walk on the top	32x		
	1-16	straddle down right alternating straddle	3x 1x	alternately: 1,2: overhead press; 3, 4: chest press	4x
	1-16	straddle down left alternating straddle	3x 1x	alternately: 1,2: overhead press; 3, 4: chest press	4x
	1-32	side lunge alternately right and left (starting on the right foot)	8x	diagonal punch	16x
	1-32	lunge back alternately right and left (starting on the right foot)	8x	rowing arms	16x
	1-8	straddle down right alternating straddle	1x 1x	alternately: 1,2: overhead press; 3, 4: chest press	2x
	1-8	straddle down left alternating straddle	1x 1x	alternately: 1,2: overhead press; 3, 4: chest press	2x
	1-16	side lunge alternately right and left (starting on the right foot)	4x	diagonal punch	8x
	1-16	lunge back alternately right and left (starting on the right foot)	4x	rowing arms	8x
	1-8	alternating straddle (r/l.)	2x	altern.: 1,2: overh. press	2x
	1-4	side lunge alternately right and left	1x	diagonal punch	2x
	1-4	lunge back alternately right and left	1x	rowing arms	2x
Elemen D	1-32	walk on the top	32x		
	1-32	basic step (down down up up) right foot leads	8x		
	1-32	basic step	8x	biceps curl (both arms)	16x
	1-16	basic step	4x	biceps curl (both arms)	
	1-16	basic step	4x		8x

Element					
Element	1-32	walk on the top	32x		
A+B+C+D	1-32	straddle down right		alternately: 1,2: overhead	8x
		alternating straddle	8x	press; 3, 4: chest press	
	1-32	side lunge alternately	8x	diagonal punch	16x
		right and left (starting			
		on the right foot)			
	1-32	lunge back alternately	8x	rowing arms	16x
		right and left (starting			
		on the right foot)			
	1-32	basic step right	7x	biceps curl (both arms)	16x
		alternating step	1x		
	1-32	walk on the top			
		now the leading leg is changed			
	1-32	straddle down left	8x	alternately: 1,2: overhead	8x
		alternating straddle		press; 3, 4: chest press	
	1-32	side lunge alternately	8x	diagonal punch	16x
		left and right (starting			
		on the left foot)			
	1-32	lunge back alternately	8x	rowing arms	16x
		left and right (starting			
		on the left foot)			
	1-32	basic step left	7x	biceps curl (both arms)	16x
		alternating step	1x		
	1-32	walk on the top			
		followed by the original combination			
	1-16	straddle down (starting	4x	alternately: 1,2: overhead	4x
		on the right foot)		press; 3, 4: chest press	
	1-16	side lunge alternately	4x	diagonal punch	8x
		right and left (starting			
		on the right foot)			
	1-16	lunge back alternately	4x	rowing arms	8x
		right and left (starting			
		with the right)			
	1-16	basic step right	3x	biceps curl (both arms)	8x
		alternating step with			
		tap to a count of 4	1x		
	1-16	straddle down (starting	4x	alternately: 1,2: overhead	4x
		on the left foot)		press; 3, 4: chest press	
	1-16	side lunge alternately	4x	diagonal punch	8x
		left and right (starting			
		on the left foot)			

| | 1-16 | lunge back alternately left and right (starting on the left foot) | 4x | rowing arms | 8x |
| | 1-16 | basic step left alternating step with tap to a count of 4 | 3x
1x | biceps curl (both arms) | 8x |

Choreography 7

Target group: Advanced –
Emphasis: dancing/co-ordinative

Elements	Cnts.	Pos. at the step	Leg movements	Rpts.	Arm movements	Rpts.
Element A	1-8		V-step	2x	a combination of chest press with rowing arms	2x
	1-8		Pony step (only to the right); on the 2nd pony step, to a count of 3+4 down tap	2x	rolling arms	8x
	1-8		V-step (first left, then right)	2x	a combination of chest press with rowing arms	2x
	1-8		Pony step (only to the left); on the 2nd pony step, to a count of 3+4 down tap	2x	rolling arms	2x
Element B	1-8		repeat knee lift step with a quarter turn around the left shoulder out and the right shoulder back. 1. kn. lift on the spot 2. turn 3. turn back	1x	walking arms	8x
	1-4		reverse turn step (left foot starts)	1x	let the arms swing loosely	1x

	1-4		Jumping Jack (at the right end of the step)	2x	deltoid arms	2x
	1-8		repeat knee lift step with a quarter turn round the right shoulder out and the left shoulder back 1. kn. lift on the spot 2. turn 3. turn back	1x	walking arms	8x
	1-4		reverse turn step (right foot starts)	1x	let the arms swing loosely	
	1-4		Jumping Jack (on the 2nd Jumping Jack jump an eighth of a turn to the left)	2x	deltoid arms	2x
Element C	1-2		tap up – tap down (right foot starts)	1x	pumping arms	2x
	1-4		Charleston step (right foot starts)	1x	walking arms	4x
	1-2		take a step forward with the right foot and jump 1/2 – 3/4 of a turn round the left shoulder	1x		
	1-8		turn step (left)	2x	semicircle arms	2x
	1-2		tap up – tap down	1x	pumping arms	2x
	1-4		Charleston step	1x	walking arms	4x
	1-2		take a step forward with the left foot and jump			

	1-8		1/2 – 3/4 of a turn round the right shoulder turn step (right)	2x	semicircle arms	
Element D	1-4	l.\ r.	kick ball, change step with a 1/4 of a turn round the left shoulder	1x	arms on the waist, clap hands to a count of 4	
	1-4	1 2	kick ball, change step with a 1/4 of a turn round the left shoulder (right starts)	1x	arms on the waist, clap hands to a count of 4	
	1-4		Piqué jump step (starting right out and left back)	2x	circle arms	2x
	1-4		kick ball change straddle step (right foot starts)	1x	arms on the waist, clap hands to a count of 4	
	1-4	1 2	kick ball change step with a 1/4 of a turn round the left shoulder (right starts)	2x	arms on the waist, clap hands to a count of 4	
	1-8		Piqué jump step (starting right out and left back)	1x	circle arms	2x

Choreography 8

Target group: Advanced – Emphasis: dancing/co-ordinative

Blocks	Elements	Cnts.	Position at the step	Leg movements	Rpts.	Arm movements	Rpts.
Block A (to the left) 1-16	Element A (to the left)	1-8		2 L-pattern (High-Impact)	2x	clap hands	4x
	Element B (to the left)	1-4		1 Charleston kick step	2x	boxing arms	4x
	Element C (to the left)	5, 6		180° turn to the right 180° turn to the left		hands on the waist	
	Element D	7		squat right		funky arms	
		8		pull left to right		clap hands	
Block B (like Block A) (to the right) 1-16	Element A (to the right)	1-8	as above, starting with left foot				
	Element B (to the right)	1-4	as above, starting with left foot				
	Element C (to the right)	5, 6	as above, do a 180° turn starting with the left foot				
	Element D	7	squat left				
		8	pull right to left				
Block C 1-16	Element A	1-4		kick ball change straddle step (starting on the right foot)	1x	walking arms	3x
		auf 4				double clap hands	1x
	Element B	5-8		kick ball change with a 1/4 turn to the left	1x	walking arms	3x
		auf 4				double clap hands	1x
	Element C	1-4		Piqué jump to the right with 1/2 a turn to the right	1x	circle arms outwards	1x
	Element D	5-8		Piqué jump to the right with 3/4 a turn to the left	1x	circle arms outwards	1x

Block	Element	1-4		as above, kick ball change straddle step (starting on the right foot)
D (like	A			
Block	Element	5-8		as above, kick ball change with a quarter of a turn to the left
C)	B			
1-16	Element	1-4		as above, Piqué jump on the right foot with 1/2 a turn to the right
	C			
	Element	5-8		as above, Piqué jump on the left foot with 3/4 of a turn to the left, returning to the starting
	D			

Choreographic instruction

Blocks	Elements	Cnts.	Leg movements	Rpts.	Arm movements	Rpts.
		1-12	up right, tap left, down left, tap right	3x	hands on waist	
		13-16	up right, tap left, down, down	1x	hands on waist	8x
		1-12	up left, tap right, right down, tap left	3x	every time	
		13-16	up left, tap right, down, down	1x	tap clap hands	
		1-16	as above but the high-impact variation (jump)			
		1-16	as above but the high-impact variation (jump)			
Block A	Element A	1-32	L-pattern at the left-hand end of the step (right foot starts) in high-impact variation	8x	clap hands	16x
		32,33	down, down, changing sides to the right-hand end of the step (this passage is also called "bridge")			
	Element A	1-32	L-pattern at the right-hand end of the step (left leg) in high-impact variation		clap hands	16x
	Element B	1-32	up-right, kick left, down, down left, back right (Charleston step)	8x	hands on waist	
					boxing arms	
		1-32	up-right, kick left, down, down left, back right (Charleston step)	8x		32x
		31,32	down, down			
	Element C	1-32	Charleston step and 180° turn jump; walk right, walk left	4x		
			Charleston step and 180° turn jump; walk right, walk left	4x	boxing arms 4x hands on waist funky arms 2x	4x

Element D	1-32		squat right, tap left, walk left, right squat left, tap right, walk right, left	8x	
Element C and D	1-8		up right, kick left, down left, back right, jump 180°, jump 180° squat right, tap left	1x	These sequences can first be performed without and then with arms
	1-8		walk left, right	8x	
Element C and D	1-8		up left, kick right, down right, back left, jump 180°, jump 180°, squat left, tap right	1x	
	1-8		walk right, left	8x	
Element C and D	1-8		up right, kick left, down left, back right, jump 180°, jump 180°, squat right, tap left	1x	2x without arms
Element C and D	1-8		up left, kick right, down right, back left, jump 180°, jump 180°, squat left, tap right	1x	
Element C and D	1-8		up right, kick left, down left, back right, jump 180°, jump 180°, squat right, tap left	1x	2x with arms
Element C and D	1-8		up left, kick right, down right, back left, jump 180°, jump 180°, squat left, tap right	1x	
	1-16		Block A		without arms
	1-16		Block B		without arms
	1-16		Block A		with arms
	1-16		Block B		without arms

to the front

	1-16		kick ball change to the r. foot	4x	
	1-16		kick ball change to the l. foot	4x	
	1-8		kick ball change to the r. foot	2x	
	1-8		kick ball change to the l. foot	2x	
	1-4		kick ball change to the r. foot	1x	
	1-4		kick ball change to the l. foot	1x	
	1-32		kick ball change altern. l. + r.	8x	
	1-32		kick ball change altern. l. + r.	8x	**walking arms and double clap hands**. The arm of the trainer demonstrates the movement sequence of the kick ball change straddle step
	32	1-4	kick ball change straddle step diagonally left	1x	

		32	5-8	kick ball change step	1x	
			1-8	walks on the spot	8x	
			1-4	kick ball change straddle step diagonally left	1x	
			5-8	kick ball change step	1x	
			1-8	walks on the spot	8x	
			1-4	kick ball change straddle step diagonally left	1x	
			5-8	kick ball change step	1x	
			1-8	walks on the spot	8x	walking arms and double clap hand
			1-4	kick ball change straddle step diagonally left	1x	
			5-8	kick ball change step	1x	
			1-8	walks on the spot	8x	
	1-8			walk on the spot	8x	
	1-32			Piqué jump on the right foot to the front, Piqué jump on the left foot to the front alternately	8x	
	1-32			Piqué jump on the right foot to the front, Piqué jump on the left foot to the front alternately	8x	arms circle outw., whilst the trainer demonstrates the Piqué jump over the step with 1/2 a turn
	1-32			Piqué jump right with 1/2 a turn; Piqué jump left with 1/2 a turn alternately	8x	without arms
	1-32			Piqué jump right with 1/2 a turn; Piqué jump left with 1/2 a turn alternately	8x	arms circling outwards	8x
	1-8			walk on the spot	8x	walking arms
	1-32			Combine blocks C and D		without arms
	1-32			Combine blocks C and D		with arms
	1-64			Combine blocks A-D		without arms
	1-64			Combine blocks A-D		with arms

Choreography 9

Expert combination (sporting/athletic)　　Crossways step

Elements	Cnts.	Pos. at the step	Leg movements	Rpts.	Arm movements	Rpts.
Element A	1-12		V-step alternately right and left (starting with the right foot)	3x	rowing arms	3x
	13-16	starting position 1 / final position 2	flying step with 1/2 a turn round the right shoulder	1x / 3x	circle arms backwards	1x / 3x
	1-12		V-step alternately right and left (starting with the right foot)	3x	rowing arms	3x
	13-16	starting position 1-4 / final position	flying step with 1/2 a turn round the right shoulder	1x / 3x	circle arms backwards	1x / 3x
Element B	1-12		V-step alternately left and right (starting with the left foot)	3x	rowing arms	3x
	13-16	starting position 1 / final position 2	flying step with 1/2 a turn round the left shoulder	1x / 3x	circle arms backwards	1x / 3x
	1-12		V-step alternately left and right (starting with the left foot)	3x	rowing arms	3x
	13-16	starting position 1 / final position 2	flying step with 1/2 a turn round the left shoulder	1x	circle arms backwards	1x

Element C	1-12		basic step	3x	shoulder pulls	6x
	13-16		Jumping Jack	2x	deltoid arms	2x
	1-12		basic step	3x	shoulder pulls	6x
	13-16		Jumping Jack	2x	deltoid arms	2x
Element D	1-12		basic step	3x	shoulder pulls	6x
	13-16		Jumping Jack	2x	deltoid arms	2x
	1-12		basic step	3x	shoulder pulls	6x
	13-16		Jumping Jack (on the second Jack turn to the 1/4 turn to the right)	2x	deltoid arms	2x
Element E	1-12		up & over	3x	circle arms	3x
	13-16		Jumping Jack (with two 1/4 turns during the Jacks round the left shoulder)	2x	lateral raises	2x
	1-12		up & over	3x	circle arms	3x
	13-16		Jumping Jack (with two 1/4 turns during the Jacks round the left shoulder)	2x	lateral raises	2x
Element F	1-8		repeat diagonally on the right foot with knee lift (2), side lift (4), hamstring curl (6) (down, down with a 1/4 of a turn to the left)	1x	**combined** chest press (2), triceps kick side (4), kick back (6) and overhead press to a count of 7, 8	1x

	1-8		repeat diagonally on the left foot with knee lift (2), side lift (4), hamstring curl (6) (down, down with a 1/4 of a turn to the right)	1x	**combined** chest press (2), triceps kick side (4), kick back (6) and overhead press to a count of 7, 8	1x
	1-8		repeat diagonally on the right foot with knee lift (2), side lift (4), hamstring curl (6) (down, down with a 1/4 of a turn to the left)	1x	**combined** chest press (2), butterfly (4), rowing arms (6) and overhead press to a count of 7, 8	1x
	1-8		repeat diagonally on the left foot with knee lift (2), side lift (4), hamstring curl (6) (down, down with a 1/4 of a turn to the right)	1x	**combined** chest press (2), butterfly (4), rowing arms (6) and overhead press to a count of 7, 8	1x

Choreography 10

Target group: Experts
Emphasis: dancing–co-ordinative   Long step

Elements	Cnts.	Positions at the step	Leg Movements	Rpts.	Arm Movements	Rpts.
Element A	1-2		up right, knee lift left (jumped)	1x	lateral pull	1x
	3-4		touch left, side lift left (jumped) and coming forward a little with the right foot	1x	deltoid arms	1x
	5-6		touch left, knee lift left (jumped) and coming forward a little with the right foot	1x	lateral pull	1x
	7-8		straddle down (left foot starts)	1x	pumping arms	2x
	1-2		up left, knee lift right (jumped)	1x	lateral pull	1x

	3-4		touch right, side lift right (jumped) and going back a little with the left foot	1x	deltoid arms	1x
	5-6		touch right, knee lift right (jumped) and going back a little with the left foot.	1x	lateral pull	1x
	7-8		straddle down (right foot starts).	1x	pumping arms	2x
Element B	1-4		corner to corner (right foot starts/ r. (1), l. (2), r. (3), l. (4)	1x	circle arms	1x
	5-8		touch left (1), touch left (2), bounce step with 1/2 a turn round the left shoulder	1x	to a cnt. of 1+2 pushing arms with l. foot, to a cnt. of 3+4 let the arms swing in time	1x
	9-12		reverse turn step (right foot starts)	1x	butterfly arms	1x
	13-16		up & over	1x	circle arms	1x
	1-4		corner to corner	1x	circle arms	1x
	5-8		touch right (1), touch right (2), bounce step with 1/2 a turn round the right shoulder	1x	to a cnt. of 1+2 pushing arms with r. foot, to a cnt. of 3+4 let the arms swing in time	1x
	9-12		reverse turn step (left foot starts)	1x	butterfly arms	1x
	13-16		up & over	1x	circle arms	1x
Element C	1-4		L-pattern	1x	pumping arms	2x
	5-6		straddle down	1x	walking arms	2x
	7-8		jump on the top and bounce	1x	pumping arms	2x

	9-10		squat to the right	1x	right hand slaps the right thigh	1x
	11-12		squat to the left	1x	left hand slaps the left thigh	1x
	13-14		legs remain on the spot in Plié		shake your body	
	15-16		jump on the top and bounce	1x	pumping arms	2x
	1-2		squat to the right	1x	right hand slaps the right thigh	1x
	3-4		squat to the left	1x	left hand slaps the left thigh	1x
	5-6		legs remain on the spot in Plié		shake your body	
	7-8		jump on the top and bounce	1x	pumping arms	2x
	9-10		straddle down (right foot starts).	1x	walking arms	2x
	11-12		step back	2x	walking arms	2x
	13-14		L-pattern	1x	pumping arms	2x
Element D	1-8		top lunge to the right	1x	to a count of 1+2 pumping arms, to a count of 3-6 diagonal punch, to a count of 7+8 pumping arms	2x 2x 2x
	1-8		top lunge to the left	1x	to a count of 1+2 pumping arms, to a count of 3-6 diagonal punch, to a count of 7+8 pumping arms	2x 2x 2x

	1-8		top lunge to the right	1x	to a count of 1+2 pumping arms,	2x
					to a count of 3-6 diagonal punch,	2x
					to a count of 7+8 pumping arms	2x
	1-8		top lunge to the left	1x	to a count of 1+2 pumping arms,	2x
					to a count of 3-6 diagonal punch,	2x
					to a count of 7+8 pumping arms	2x

5.4 Phase: Walk-down

Example: *Walk-down*

Counts	Leg movements	Rpts.	Arm movement	Rpts.
1-14	walk on the top (right foot leads)	14x	walking arms	
15-16	down right, tap left		walking arms	
1-14	walk on the top (left foot leads)	14x	walking arms	
15-16	down left, tap right		walking arms	
1-6	walk on the top (right foot leads)	6x	walking arms	
7-8	down right, tap left		walking arms	
1-6	walk on the top (left foot leads)	6x	walking arms	
7-8	down left, tap right		walking arms	
1-16	alternating step with tap to a count of 4	4x	walking arms	
1-32	alternating step with tap to a count of 2	8x	shake arms out to the side	
1-16	tap up right, down left, tap up left, down right	8x	snap your fingers	
1-16	flex up right, down right, flex up left, down left	8x	circle arms to the side	2x
1-16	kick to the right and left with a repeat in front of the step	8x	shake the arms out in front of you	
1-16	kick to the right and left with a repeat in front of the step	8x	shake the arms out whilst lifting them to a count of 4 and then bringing them down again to a count of 4	2x
1-32	step touch	16x	swinging arms	

5.5 Phase: Floor Workout

We will now give two examples of muscle power training, including the exercises, sequences as well as the degree of exertion and number of repeats. The information first looks at a power-training programme for beginners, but also one for the more advanced. We give levels of stress for your own judgement.

Muscle trembling and incorrect performance of an exercise are clear indications that one should take a breath. The main criterion here is to adjust stress level in accordance with a subjective sense of exertion.

Example: Beginners

Muscle group	Exercise	Repeat	No. of movem.
Buttocks	Bench position at the long side of the step, supporting the lower arms on the step and bending the left leg at knee and ankle to 90°. Then raise and lower the bent leg in small movements.	each leg alternately 16x	2-3x
Back	Bench position at the long side of the step, supporting the lower arms on the step. Stretch the right arm and left leg, moving then underneath the body, alternately right and left.	16x	2-3x
Back	Lying on one's tummy along the step, with the thighs on the ground, the forehead on the step platform and the arms stretched upwards. Take the arms round the side to the back and then back to the starting position.	16x	2-3x
Right abductors	Lying on the side of the body across the step apparatus with the upper leg bent on the step. Move your leg off the platform and raise and lower it in small movements. Roll on your tummy over the step platform to the other side.		
Left abductors	as above	16x Repeat 2-3 x	1x
Straight tummy	Lying on your back along the step, press both feet at the heels firmly into the platform, keeping both hands on the temples. Roll up the upper body and lower it.	16x	2-3x
Transverse stomach muscles	Lying on your back along the step, press both feet at the heels firmly into the platform; put your right hand behind your head and take your left arm diagonally towards the right knee. Roll up the upper body diagonally and lower it.	16x	2x

Example: Advanced and experts

Muscle group	Exercise	Repeat	No. of movem.
Back	Lying on your stomach along the step, head and chest are raised from the platform, and arms held to the side of the body turned towards the outside. Finally, the upper body is lowered and the arms turned in.	16-24x	3-4x
Buttocks	From the bench position, the right/ left leg is bent 90° at the knee and ankle. The leg is raised and lowered with very little movement.	16-24x	3-4x
Rear thigh	From the bench position, the right/ left leg is stretched. The heel is pulled towards the buttocks and back again.	16-24x	3-4x
Chest	Lying on your back along the step with legs drawn up, the arms are brought from the side to the front. To increase intensity use hand weights or Thera Bands.	16-24x	3-4x
Stomach	Lying on your back along the step, the arms are lifted up and one arm is bent at the elbow. The upper body is rolled up and then lowered. The position is maintained while the upper body is rolled up and lowered alternately, diagonally to the left and diagonally to the right.	16-24x	3-4x

5.6 Phase: Cool-down

Example: Cool-down

Counts	Leg movements	Rpts.	Arm movement	Rpts.
1-32	walking on the spot	32x	shaking arms out in all directions	32x
1-32	step touch	16x	circle arms round high to the side, breathing in and out deeply	4x
1-16	step kick	8x	snap your fingers	8x
1-16	step touch	8x	clap hands	8x
1-32	double side step	8x	combined snapping fingers and clapping hands	8x
1-32	grapevine step	8x	circle arms (swinging them loosely)	8x
1-16	turn step through 360° (alternately to l. and r.)	4x	let your arms swing loosely at the side of your body.	4x
1-16	step touch	8x		
1-16	side to side	8x	no arms	–
1-16	side to side	8x	swinging arms	8x
1-16	step touch	8x	shake out the arms from low down at the front, upwards and then down again.	2x (1 movem. = 8 counts)
1-16	bounce	16x	swinging arms	8x

It is also appropriate to use the classic cool-down alongside stretching and relaxation exercises when in the relaxation phase.

Stepped resting

Cab driver's position

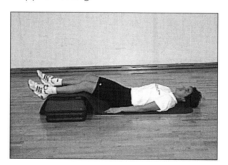
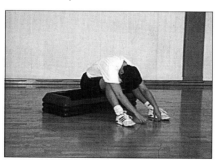

6   *Ideas for Schools*

In this chapter, we will present two lesson plans for sessions with older pupils. As an example, two 90-minute units are worked on which concentrate on training general dynamic endurance and strength. The suggestions are to be taken as possible alternatives to the usual school sport fitness training.

The lack of standardised step apparatus should not prevent teachers from using step training. There is a wide range of traditional gymnastic apparatus which can be turned into a step platform. Gymnastic mats piled on top of each other have proved well-suited for the job, but also jumping boards pushed into each other and the upper sections of large gymnastic boxes will work (see Chapter 1).

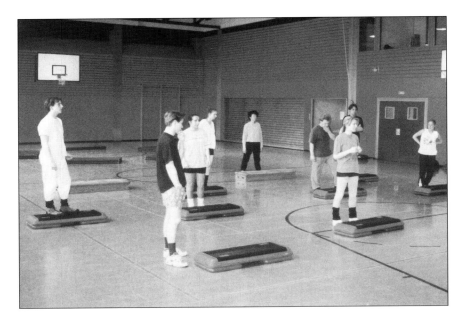

Action with pupils

Lesson plan 1:
Emphasis on training general aerobic endurance

As detailed below, we start with a 90-minute lesson unit. As far as the contents are concerned, classic aerobics training is covered in the first part of the lesson. This training follows a similar procedure that is used in fitness studios. A step-specific warm-up follows the normal warm-up and stretching, and then comes the actual endurance phase, the choreography. This individual training gives way to variations with a partner as well as group formation in the second part. Before any training takes place with and at the step apparatus, the pupils should be given a theoretical briefing of what body posture is all about during step aerobics, as well as safety precautions at the step:

- take up a starting position about 20 cm away from the step,
- always put the whole sole of your foot in the middle of the platform,
- knee and foot should always be in line with each other,
- the main body muscles should be tightly tensed, as the whole body is lent forwards towards the step from the sole of one's foot,
- turns may only be done on the non-load-bearing leg.

Lesson part 1: Individual Training

Apparatus: Step apparatus, upper section of gymnastics box or gymnastics mats.
Starting position: one pupil per step with all pupils facing to the front.

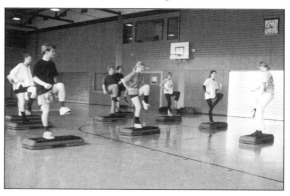

Starting position front

Phase: Warm-up

Cnts	Leg movements	Rpts.	Arm movement	Rpts.
1-8	walk on the spot (walking steps)	1x		
1-8	walk on the spot	3x	arms circling over the shoulder to the hips, breathe in, arms circling over the hips to the shoulders, breathe out	3x 3x
1-8	walk on the spot	3x	spread out the hands alternately, punch your arms to the side, circling high and low	3x 3x
1-8	walk on the spot	1x	shake out your arms	
1-8	step right, left, right, left, tap (tap up) step left, right, left, right, tap (alternating step)	2x		
1-8	-"-	2x	clap hands to the tap	2x
1-8	step right forw., l. to the side, r. to the middle back, r. tap step l. forwards, r. to the side, l. to the middle, r. tap (= 2 V-steps)	2x		
1-8	2 V-steps	2x	clap to tap	2x
1-8	step r., l., r., l., tap, step l., r., l., r., tap (alternating step)	2x	snap fingers to the tap	
1-8	step r. forw., l. sidew., r. back with 1/4 of a turn r., l. tap; step l. sidew., r. forw., sidew. on 1/4 of a turn l., l. backw. on 1/4 of a turn l., r. tap (= 2 turn step)	2x		
1-8	2 turn step	2x	whilst the right, then the left arm does a circle at chest height; clap to the tap	
1-8	walk on the spot (with 1/4 of a turn right to the front)	1x	walking arms	8x
1-8	4 steps forw., 4 steps backw.	2x	circle arms forw. whilst walking backw.; circle arms backw. whilst walking forw.	2x
1-8	8 steps on the spot side step right, left tap and side step left, right tap (=step touch)	1x 4x	walking arms	8x
1-8	double side step	2x		
1-8	step to the r., l. cross backw., r. side, l. tap; step to the l., r. cross backw., l. side, r. tap (=grapevine)	2x		
1-8	grapevine	2x	lift arms to shoulder level and then lower	8x

1-8	walk on the spot (walk in)	1x	
1-8	walk on the spot with legs open (=walk out)	1x	
1-8	walk in	1x	
1-8	walk out	1x	
1-8	in small knee bends in walk-out position (=Plié)	2x	
1-8	do plié movement in walk-out position	2x	lower arms bent tow. the body from the elbow (biceps curl)

Phase: Stretching

Muscles used	Description of exercise
Lower right thigh muscle	Transfer weight onto the left leg from the Plié position; stretch the right leg out with ankle bent and tilt the upper body forwards keeping the back straight.
Front right thigh muscle	Roll up the upper body, then pull your right heel towards your right buttock with your right hand.
Right calf muscle	Bend the left leg putting the right leg back in striding position; press the right heel into the ground.
Inner right thigh muscle	Turn your upper body a 1/4 of a turn to the right, keeping your left leg in plié; bend your back straight forwards, pressing the right outstretched leg into the ground flexing the foot.
Right hip bender	Turn the upper body a 1/4 of a turn to the left, putting it then on the left thigh; both hands rest on the floor with the right leg placed well backwards.
	Bring the right leg towards the left leg and roll the upper body up slowly.
	Now repeat all the stretching exercises for the left side of the body.

Phase: Warm-up step-specific

Cnts	Leg movements	Rpts.	Arm movement	Rpts.
1-8	walk in front of the step to a count of 4 left, tap on the step walks in front of the step, to a count of 4 right, tap on the step	4x		
1-8	r. up, l. up, r. down, l. tap down l. up, r. up, l. down, r. tap down (= alternating)	4x		
1-8	8 steps on the step, starting with the right foot	1x		
1-8	8 steps in front of the step	1x		

1-8	4 steps on the step, 4 steps in front of the step	2x		
1-8	alternating: 2 steps on the step, 2 steps in front of the step	4x		
1-8	8 steps on the step starting with the left foot	1x		
1-8	8 steps in front of the step	1x		
1-8	4 steps on the step, 4 steps in front of the step	2x		
1-8	alternating: 2 steps on the step, 2 steps in front of the step	4x		
1-8	r. up, l. tap, l. down, r. down l. up, r. tap, r. down, l. down	4x		
1-8	r. up, l. knee lift, l. down, r. down, l. up, r. knee lift, r. down, l. down	4x		

Phase: Choreography

Cnts	Leg movements	Rpts.	Arm movement	Rpts.
1-8	2 V-steps right and left	4x		
1-8	2 V-steps right and left	4x	chest press	16x
1-8	alternating step right and left	4x		
1-8	r. up (r. end of step), l. up (l. end of step), r. down, back, l. tap l. up (l. end of step), r. up (r. end of step), l. down, back, r. tap	4x		
1-8	2 turn steps	4x		
1-8	2 turn steps	4x	semi circle arms	8x
	We now stand with our right shoulder to the step			
1-8	r. up, l. tap, l. down, r. tap r. up, l. tap, l. down, r. tap	2x		
1-8	Twice up & over	2x		
1-8	Twice up & over	4x	circle arms	8x
1-8	up r., l. tap, l. down, r. tap up r., l. tap, l. down, r. tap	2x		
1-8	up r., l. knee lift, l. down, r. tap up r., l. knee lift, l. down, r. tap	2x		
1-8	knee lift diagonally; after the fourth knee lift to a count of 15/16, 1/2 a turn to the right, so that the diagonal changes	2x		
1-8	up l., r. tap, r. down, l. tap up l., r. tap, r. down, l. tap	2x		
1-8	up l., r. knee l., r. down, l. tap up l., r. knee l., r. down, l. tap	2x		

1-8	knee lift diagonally	2x		
1-8	knee lift steps diagonally r. and l.	4x		
1-8	knee lift steps diagonally r. and l. (during the 8 repeats, the verbal instruction or V-step is given)	4x	overhead press arms	16x
1-8	2 V-steps	2x		
	2 V-steps	2x	chest press	8x
1-8	2 turn steps	2x		
1-8	2 turn steps	2x	semi-circle arms	4x
1-8	2 up & over starting with the r. foot	2x		
1-8	2 up & over	2x	circle arms	4x
1-8	2 knee lift steps diagonally	2x		
1-8	2 knee lift steps diagonally	2x	overhead press arms	8x
Each element is done to a count of 8 (choreography)				
1-8	2 V-steps	1x	chest press	4x
1-8	2 turn steps	1x	semi-circle arms	2x
1-8	2 up & over	1x	circle arms	2x
1-8	knee lift diagonally	1x	overhead press	4x

Still continuing to train the general skills of performance potential, the number of repeats can be varied as follows:

Lesson part 2: Variations with a partner and a group

1. Step choreography by working in pairs:
Apparatus: 2 gymnastic mats on top of each other per pair.
Starting position: each pair of pupils stands opposite each other at the long side of the mats.
Doing the exercise: the choreography is performed as before but during the elements "V-step with chest press" and "turn-step with semi-circle arms" the partners may touch each others' palms.

2. Step choreography in group formation:
Apparatus: 2 mats on top of each other per pair placed in a circle.
Starting position: 2 pupils per mat stand opposite each other at the long side of the mats.

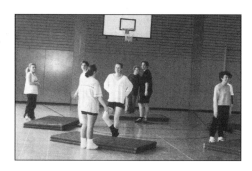

Mat circle

Doing the exercise:
The choreography is done once to 64 counts (i.e. each of the 4 elements is performed 4 times). The fourth element of the choreography, however, is only repeated twice, because the pupils swap over to the next mat doing 8 steps to the final 8 counts. Then the choreography is repeated with a new partner.

Lesson plan 2:
Emphasis on training strength skills

Lesson structure

The structure of a lesson where strength skills are emphasized runs as follows: during the first part of the lesson, the individual training of the previous lesson is repeated. Warm-up, stretch, step-specific warm-up and the choreography are therefore identical.

After that sequence come functional exercises for strengthening the back muscles, the leg muscles and the tummy muscles. This floor-work phase concludes with a cool-down.

The strengthening exercises of the floor-work phase are done using step apparatus or similar arrangements of apparatus. The following performances describe the various exercises in detail, ending with a short explanation of the methods involved.

Strength exercises with the step

Exercise 1
Muscles: Upper section of back muscles
Starting position: lying on your tummy along the step with your thighs on the ground and forehead on the step platform, the arms are then bent to the side. *Doing the exercise:*
raise both arms simultaneously to shoulder level and then lower them again.

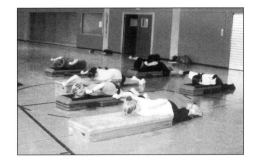

• • • • •

Variation: move the arms forwards and backwards whilst they are at shoulder level.

Exercise 2
Muscles: Back muscles
Starting position: Bench-position at the short side of the step, supporting the lower arms on the step, stretch the right arm and left leg.
Doing the exercise:
pull the right elbow and left knee under the body simultaneously finishing with stretching.
Variation: the stretched extremities of the body are moved up and down with very little movement.

Exercise 3
Muscles: Chest muscles
Starting position: press-ups at the short side of the step with both hands on the step.
Doing the exercise: simultaneously bend and stretch the arms (press-ups).

Exercise 4
Muscles: Arm muscles
Starting position: sitting on the long side of the step with the soles of your feet well away from your body, support yourself on your hands at the side of your body.
Doing the exercise:
take your buttocks off the step and alter the body's centre of gravity, pressing it down and 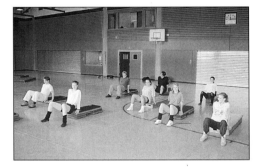 pushing it up by bending and stretching your arms.

Exercise 5
Muscles: Stomach muscles
Starting position: lying on your back beside the long side of the step, put both feet on the step platform and cross your arms over your chest.
Doing the exercise:
roll your body up diagonally and then lower it (curl).

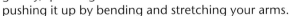

• • • • •

Exercise 6
Muscles: Leg muscles
Starting position: lying on your side beside the long side of the step, with your upper leg bent onto the step.
Doing the exercise: raise your other leg from the ground and raise and lower it with very little movement.

Methodic procedure

Basically, when planning the sequence of exercises, one should take care that the exercises flow smoothly into one another. The methodic principles of the endurance phase can be transferred to the floor-work. A good example of this is the exercise for strengthening the upper back. One can look back to the example of an "upturned pyramid" (within the technique section) or the correct method.

Diagram 7: Methodic sequence for the exercise: strengthening the upper back

Cnts:	Movement	Repeats
1-32	lower both arms and raise them to shoulder level. (Movement A)	8x
1-32	push forward and then pull back the arms, keeping them at shoulder level. (Movement B)	8x
1-16	Movement A	4x
1-16	Movement B	4x
1-8	Movement A	2x
1-8	Movement B	2x
1-8	Movement A	2x
1-8	Movement B	2x

7 Bibliography

ABELE, A./ BREHM, W.: Mood Effects of Exercise versus Sports Games: Findings and Implications for Well-being and Health. In: International Review of Health Psychology (1993), 53-80.

BALZ, E./ BRINKHOFF, K.P./ WEGNER, U.: Neue Sportarten in die Schule! In: Sportpädagogik 18 (1994), 2, 17-14.

BAUR, C.: Step-Aerobic. In: UHLIG, T. (Hrsg.): Gesundheitssport im Verein. Schorndorf 1995, 161-166.

BOECKH-BEHRENS, W.-U./ BUSKIES, W.: Gesundheitsorientiertes Fitneß-training. Bd. 1. Lüneburg 1995.

BORG, G.: An Introduction to Borg's RPE-scale. Ithaca 1985.

BREHM, W.: Fitneß – ein großer Renner ohne die Schule. Vortragsmanuskript zum 1. Kongreß des Deutschen Sportlehrerverbandes in Leipzig. Universität Bayreuth 1995.

BREHM, W.: Im Augenblick aufgehen – Emotionales Erleben bei (Step-) Aerobic und anderen Fitneßaktivitäten. Vortragsmanuskript zur 9. Bodylife Fachtagung in Karlsruhe. Universität Bayreuth 1995.

BREHM, W./ PAHMEIER, I.: Gesundheitsförderung durch sportliche Aktivierung als gemeinsame Aufgabe von Ärzten, Krankenkassen und Sportvereinen. Bielefeld 1992.

BREHM, W./ PAHMEIER, I./ TIEMANN, M.: Gesundheitsförderung durch sportliche Aktivierung. Projektbericht Band 1. Universität Bayreuth 1994.

BRETTSCHNEIDER, W. D./ BRÄUTIGAM, M.: Sport in der Alltagswelt von Jugendlichen. Forschungsbericht. Düsseldorf (Kultusministerium NRW) 1990.

BUSKIES, W./ BENKER, A./ BOECKH-BEHRENS, W.-U./ ZIESCHANG, K.: Zur Problematik der metabolischen und kardialen Belastung bei zwei verschiedenen Krafttrainingsmethoden. In: Liesen, H. M./ Weiss, M./ Baum (Hrsg.): Regulations- und Repairmechanismen. 33. Dt. Sportärztekongreß. Köln 1994, 97-99.

BUSKIES, W./ KLÄGER, G./ RIEDEL, H.: Möglichkeiten zur Steuerung der Belastungsintensität für ein breitensportlich orientiertes Laufausdauertraining. In: Deutsche Zeitschrift für Sportmedizin 43 (1992), 248-260.

DE MAREES, H.: Sportphysiologie. Schriftenreihe von den Troponwerken. Köln/ Mühlheim 1987.

DT. AEROBIC VERBAND E.V. (Hrsg.): Aerobic. Bonn 1993.

DTB (Hrsg.): Aerobic als Gesundheitssport. Frankfurt/ Main 1993.

DTB (Hrsg.): Broschüre Allgemeines Turnen 1996. Frankfurt/ Main 1995.

DTB (Hrsg.): Step-Aerobic. Frankfurt/ Main 1994.

FONDA, J.: Jane-Fondas Fitneß-Buch. „Ich fühle mich gut!". Frankfurt/ Main 1983.

FOX, M.: Step on It. New York 1991

FREIWALD, J.: Fitneß für Männer. Reinbek 1991.

FREYTAG-BAUMGARTNER, M.: Aerobics. Niedernhausen 1994.

FRIEDRICH, M.: Attraktion der Step-Aerobic! Diplomarbeit. Universität Bayreuth 1995.

GROOS, E./ ROTHMAIER, D.: Ausdauergymnastik.
Neue Aerobics von 20 bis 70. Reinbek bei Hamburg 1991.

HEINEMANN, K./ SCHUBERT, M.: Der Sportverein. Ergebnisse einer repräsentativen Untersuchung. Schorndorf 1994.

HOLLMANN, W./ HETTINGER, T.: Sportmedizin. 3., durchges. Auflage Stuttgart, New York 1990.

INSTITUT FÜR FREIZEITWIRTSCHAFT: Wachstumsfelder im Freizeit und Tourismusbereich, Teil 9: Sport. München 1993.

JOHNSON, V.: Victoria Johnson's Attitude. Hamondsworth, England 1993.

KAMBEROVIC, R./ HASE, T.: Fitneß & Profit. Wedel 1994.

KNEBEL, K.-P.: Funktionsgymnastik. Reinbek b. Hamburg 1994.

KOBUSCH-NIEDERBÄUMER, C.: Step-Aerobic – Eine empirische Beanspruchungsanalyse. Diplomarbeit, Universität Bielefeld 1994.

KREMPEL, O.: Anti Cellulite Training. Reinbek bei Hamburg 1994.

LAGERSTROEM, D.: Fitneßtraining. In: Lagerstroem, D./ Völker, K. (Hrsg:): Freizeitsport. Erlangen 1983, 29-44.

NIEDERBÄUMER, C./ PAHMEIER, I.: Step-Aerobic – Fitneßtraining in der Schule!?
In: Sportunterricht (1996) i.Dr.

RIEDER, H./LEHNERTZ, K.: Bewegungslernen und Techniktraining. Schorndorf 1991.

RIPPE, J.: Mit dem Step-Training in eine neue Ära! In: Bodylife (1994), 94-99.

ROME, S.: Aerobic: Bewegungstraining, das Spaß macht. 1983.

SCHULZ, N.: Mit der Zeit gehen – zur Aktualisierung von Schulsportinhalten. In: Sportunterricht 43 (1994), 12, 492-503.

SHEPPARD-MISSED, J.: Jazzexercise. California 1986.

SOERENSEN, J.: Aerobic-Dancing: Schön, schlank und fit im Rhythmus unserer Zeit. 1983.

WEINECK, J.: Optimales Training. Erlangen 1990.

WOPP; C.: Entwicklungen und Perspektiven des Freizeitsports. Aachen 1995.

Aerobic & Dance

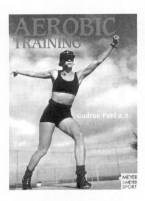

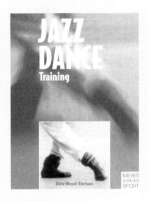

Gudrun Paul a.o.
Aerobic Training

This book deals with the general principals of fitness training, as well as those specifically belonging to aerobics.
The reader can see how to build up a series of lessons in aerobics training with many practical examples and, in particular, various basic steps and their technical application are introduced.
At the same time, ways of communication – method and cueing – are described and the book also shows many ways of varying aerobics training.

160 pages
126 photos, 16 figures
Paperback, 14.8 x 21 cm
ISBN 1-84126-021-5
£ 12.95 UK/$ 17.95 US/
$ 25.95 CDN

Dörte Wessel-Therhorn
Jazz Dance Training

In this book the author documents dance creation and jazz dance training according to the method of the renowned Swiss choreographer Alain Bernard.
The book contains a short summary of the evolution of jazz dance from its roots in folklore to its modern status as a style of performance dance. In addition, it provides descriptions of the anatomical functional basics for modern dance training and a comprehensive collection of exercises ranging from elementary to advanced.

2nd edition
208 pages
250 photos and figures
Paperback, 14.8 x 21 cm
ISBN 1-84126-041-X
£ 12.95 UK/$ 17.95 US/
$ 25.95 CDN

MEYER
& MEYER
SPORT

MEYER & MEYER Verlag | Von-Coels-Straße 390 | D-52080 Aachen, Germany | Fax + + 49 (0)2 41/9 58 10-10

Basic Fitness

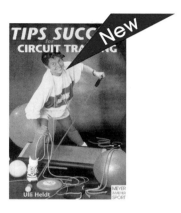

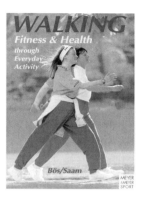

Ulli Heldt
**Tips for Success –
Circuit Training**

Remember circuit training at school? Forget it! This book presents numerous possible variations of how to make a circuit be enjoyable, interesting and effective at the same time. The main emphasis here lies on strength, endurance, co-ordination and fun. Tips for Success – Circuit Training provides all sports teachers, trainers and instructors with several new ideas for lessons with different target groups.

140 pages
Two-colour print
6 photos, 59 illustrations
Paperback, 11.5 x 18 cm
ISBN 1-84126-028-2
£ 6.95 UK/$ 9.95 US/
$ 12.95 CDN

Klaus Bös/Joachim Saam
Walking
Fitness & Health through Everyday Activity

Walking is introduced as an especially health-promoting kind of sport, which anyone can indulge in. This book describes the basics of walking technique, considers the necessary clothing, the appropriate medical background, and also gives advice on diet.
It provides interesting incentives for the professional as well as the beginner, like schemes for strengthening the whole body or tips for new kinds of walking e.g. body walking (meditative walking).

112 pages, 20 photos
Paperback, 11.5 x 18 cm
ISBN 1-84126-001-0
£ 5.95 UK/$ 8.95 US/
$ 12.95 CDN

Health

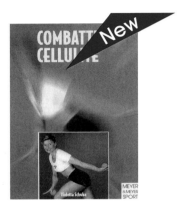

Violetta Schuba
Combatting Cellulite

This book offers a wide-ranging, practice-oriented endurance and muscle training programme alongside background information about building up one's skin, how cellulite starts and about diet. Lots of diagrams illustrate the exercise examples, which are easy to do.

144 pages
Two-colour print
70 photos and illustrations
Paperback, 14.8 x 21 cm
ISBN 1-84126-032-0
£ 9.95 UK/$ 14.95 US/
$ 20.95 CDN

MEYER
& MEYER
SPORT

If you are interested in
Meyer & Meyer Sport
and our large
programme, please
visit us **online**
or call our **Hotline** ▼

online:
▶ www.meyer-meyer-
sports.com

▶   Hotline:
++49 (0)1 80 / 5 10 11 15

We are looking
forward to your call!

Please order our catalogue!
Please order our catalogue!

MEYER & MEYER Verlag I Von-Coels-Straße 390 I D-52080 Aachen, Germany I Fax ++49 (0)2 41 / 9 58 10-10